OPHTHALMIC CLINICAL DEBATES

OPHTHALMIC CLINICAL DEBATES

Thomas A. Deutsch, M.D.
Associate Professor of Ophthalmology
Rush Medical College
Program Director in Ophthalmology
Rush-Presbyterian–St. Luke's Medical Center
Chicago, Illinois

YEAR BOOK MEDICAL PUBLISHERS, INC.
CHICAGO • LONDON • BOCA RATON

OPTOMETRY

03137156

1   2   3   4   5   6   7   8   9   0   C   R   93   92   91   90   89

Library of Congress Cataloging-in-Publication Data
Ophthalmic clinical debates.

Includes bibliographies and index.
1. Eye—Diseases and defects—Case studies.
I. Deutsch, Thomas A.   [DNLM: 1. Eye Diseases—therapy.
2. Ophthalmology—methods.   3. Vision Disorders—
therapy.   WW 100 0602]
RE69.064   1989   617.7   88-28055
ISBN 0-8151-2443-0

Sponsoring Editor: David K. Marshall
Associate Managing Editor, Manuscript Services: Deborah Thorp
Production Project Manager: Gayle Paprocki
Proofroom Manager: Shirley E. Taylor

To Rebecca: conceived
and delivered with this book.

CONTRIBUTORS _____

Richard L. Anderson, M.D.
Professor of Ophthalmology
Director of Oculoplastic, Orbital, and Oncology
    Services
Department of Ophthalmology
University of Utah Medical Center
Salt Lake City, Utah

Norman E. Byer, M.D.
Clinical Professor of Ophthalmology
School of Medicine
UCLA
Los Angeles, California

Marshall N. Cyrlin, M.D.
Assistant Clinical Professor
Michigan State University
Director, Glaucoma Service
Sinai Hospital
East Lansing, Michigan

Chandler R. Dawson, M.D.
Director, Francis I. Proctor Foundation for
    Research in Ophthalmology
Professor of Ophthalmology
University of California at San Francisco
San Francisco, California

Thomas A. Deutsch, M.D.
Associate Professor of Ophthalmology
Rush Medical College
Program Director in Ophthalmology
Rush-Presbyterian–St. Luke's Medical Center
Chicago, Illinois

Robert C. Drews, M.D.
Professor of Clinical Ophthalmology
Washington University School of Medicine
St. Louis, Missouri

Michael J. Elman, M.D.
Assistant Professor of Ophthalmology
University of Maryland School of Medicine
The Johns Hopkins University School of
    Medicine
Baltimore, Maryland

Randy J. Epstein, M.D.
Assistant Professor of Ophthalmology
Rush Medical College
Attending Physician
Rush-Presbyterian–St. Luke's Medical Center
Chicago, Illinois

Marianne E. Feitl, M.D.
Glaucoma Fellow
University of Pennsylvania
Scheie Eye Institute
Hospital of University of Pennsylvania
Philadelphia, Pennsylvania

Eugene R. Folk, M.D.
Professor of Ophthalmology
University of Illinois College of Medicine
Attending Ophthalmologist
University of Illinois Eye and Ear Infirmary
University of Illinois at Chicago
Chicago, Illinois

Bartley R. Frueh, M.D.
Professor of Ophthalmology
Director of Eye Plastic and Orbital Surgery
The University of Michigan
W. K. Kellogg Eye Center
Ann Arbor, Michigan

David J. Fuerst, M.D.
Director, Cornea and External Disease
 Service
White Memorial Medical Center
Los Angeles, California

Bruce R. Garretson, M.D.
Assistant Professor
University of Illinois Eye and Ear Infirmary
University of Illinois at Chicago
Chicago, Illinois

James Goodwin, M.D.
Director, Neuro-ophthalmology Service
Associate Professor of Clinical
 Ophthalmology and Neurology
University of Illinois Eye and Ear Infirmary
University of Illinois at Chicago
Chicago, Illinois

David L. Guyton, M.D.
Associate Professor of Ophthalmology
The Johns Hopkins University School of
 Medicine
Baltimore, Maryland

John B. Holds, M.D.
Clinical Instructor
Fellow in Oculoplastic, Orbital, and
 Oncologic Surgery
Department of Ophthalmology
University of Utah
Salt Lake City, Utah

Norman S. Jaffe, M.D.
Clinical Professor of Ophthalmology
Bascom Palmer Eye Institute
University of Miami School of Medicine
Miami, Florida

Frederick A. Jakobiec, M.D.

Professor of Clinical Ophthalmology and
    Clinical Pathology
Columbia University College of Physicians
    and Surgeons
Chairman, Department of Ophthalmology
Director of Laboratories
Manhattan Eye, Ear and Throat Hospital
New York City, New York

Henry J. Kaplan, M.D.

Professor and Chairman
Department of Ophthalmology
Washington University School of Medicine
Chief of Service
Barnes Hospital
St. Louis, Missouri

Ronald V. Keech, M.D.

Assistant Professor of Ophthalmology
University of Iowa
University of Iowa Hospitals and Clinics
Iowa City, Iowa

Lanning B. Kline, M.D.

Associate Professor of Clinical
    Ophthalmology, Neurology, and
    Neurosurgery
Combined Program in Ophthalmology
Department of Ophthalmology
Eye Foundation Hospital
University of Alabama School of Medicine
Birmingham, Alabama

Manus C. Kraff, M.D.

Clinical Professor of Ophthalmology
University of Illinois at Chicago
Chicago, Illinois

Theodore Krupin, M.D.
Professor, University of Pennsylvania
Scheie Eye Institute
Chief, Glaucoma Service
University of Pennsylvania Medical Center
Philadelphia, Pennsylvania

Marc F. Lieberman, M.D.
Assistant Professor of Ophthalmology
Stanford University School of Medicine
Director of Glaucoma Service
Stanford University Hospital
Palo Alto Veterans Administration Hospital
Stanford, California

David K. Linn, M.D., Ph.D.
Glaucoma Fellow
University of Louisville
Louisville, Kentucky

Timothy T. McMahon, O.D., F.A.A.O.
Assistant Professor of Optometry
University of Illinois College of Medicine at
    Chicago
Director, Contact Lens Service
University of Illinois Hospital
Chicago, Illinois

Benjamin Milder, M.D.
Professor of Clinical Ophthalmology
Washington University School of Medicine
Washington University Hospitals
St. Louis, Missouri

Robert A. Nozik, M.D. (A.B.)
Clinical Professor of Ophthalmology
Department of Ophthalmology
University of California at San Francisco
Research Ophthalmologist
Proctor Foundation
San Francisco, California

Robert B. Nussenblatt, M.D.

Clinical Director
National Eye Institute
National Institutes of Health
Bethesda, Maryland

R. Joseph Olk, M.D.

Assistant Professor of Clinical
  Ophthalmology
Washington University School of Medicine
Staff Ophthalmologist
Barnes Hospital
St. Louis, Missouri

David H. Orth, M.D.

Associate Professor
Department of Ophthalmology
Rush-Presbyterian–St. Luke's Medical Center
Director, Retinal Vascular Department
Ingalls Memorial Hospital
Chicago, Illinois

David J. Palmer, M.D.

Assistant Professor of Ophthalmology
Rush Medical College
Clinical Instructor of Ophthalmology
University of Chicago Pritzker School of
  Medicine
Michael Reese Hospital and Medical Center
Chicago, Illinois

Stephen C. Pollock, M.D.

Assistant Professor of Ophthalmology
Duke University Eye Center
Duke University
Durham, North Carolina

Carmen A. Puliafito, M.D.

Assistant Professor of Ophthalmology
Harvard Medical School
Assistant Professor
Division of Health Sciences and Technology
Massachusetts Institute of Technology
Director, Morse Laser Center
Massachusetts Eye and Ear Infirmary
Boston, Massachusetts

Jeffery B. Robin, M.D.

Associate Professor of Ophthalmology
Co-Director of Cornea and External Disease
  Service
University of Illinois at Chicago
Chicago, Illinois

I Rand Rodgers, M.D.

Fellow, Manhattan Eye, Ear and Throat
  Hospital
New York City, New York

Paul E. Romano, M.D.

Professor of Ophthalmology and Pediatrics
Department of Ophthalmology and Pediatrics
University of Florida College of Medicine
Director, Pediatric Ophthalmology and
  Ocular Motility
Shands Hospital
Gainesville, Florida

Jonathan B. Rubenstein, M.D.

Assistant Professor of Ophthalmology
Rush Medical College
Attending Physician
Rush-Presbyterian–St. Luke's Medical Center
Chicago, Illinois

Jon M. Ruderman, M.D.
Assistant Professor
Northwestern Medical School
Chief of Glaucoma Services
Northwestern Memorial Hospital
Chicago, Illinois

Peter J. Savino, M.D.
Professor of Ophthalmology
Thomas Jefferson University Hospital
Director, Neuro-Ophthalmology
Wills Eye Hospital
Clinical Professor of Ophthalmology
University of Pennsylvania
Philadelphia, Pennsylvania

Howard Schatz, M.D.
Clinical Professor of Ophthalmology
University of California at San Francisco
Director, Retina Research Fund of St. Mary's
   Hospital and Medical Center
San Francisco, California

William E. Scott, M.D.
Professor, University of Iowa School of
   Medicine
Director of Pediatric Ophthalmology
University of Iowa Hospitals and Clinics
Iowa City, Iowa

Robert M. Sinskey, M.D.
Associate Professor of Ophthalmology
UCLA
St. John's Hospital and Health Center
Los Angeles, California

Ronald E. Smith, M.D.
Professor of Ophthalmology
University of Southern California
Estelle Doheny Eye Institute
Los Angeles, California

Howard H. Tessler, M.D.
Associate Professor of Clinical
  Ophthalmology
University of Illinois at Chicago
Chicago, Illinois

Richard C. Troutman, M.D.,
F.A.C.S.
Clinical Professor of Ophthalmology
Professor Emeritus
Cornell Medical College
New York City, New York

Robert S. Weinberg, M.D.
Associate Professor of Ophthalmology
Virginia Commonwealth University
Medical College of Virginia
Director, Uveitis Service
Director, Cornea and External Disease
  Service
Medical College of Virginia
Richmond, Virginia

Robert N. Weinreb, M.D.
Professor and Vice Chairman
Department of Ophthalmology
University of California at San Diego
La Jolla, California

Kirk R. Wilhelmus, M.D.
Associate Professor
Department of Ophthalmology
Cullen Eye Institute
Baylor College of Medicine
Houston, Texas

Lawrence A. Yannuzzi, M.D.
Associate Professor Clinical Ophthalmology
Columbia University Medical School
Surgeon Director Ophthalmology
Director of Retinal Services
Manhattan Eye, Ear and Throat Hospital
New York City, New York

Thom J. Zimmerman, M.D., Ph.D.
Professor and Chairman
Department of Ophthalmology
Professor of Pharmacology and Toxicology
University of Louisville School of Medicine
Louisville, Kentucky

FOREWORD _____

When we risk no contradiction,
It prompts the tongue to deal in fiction.

John Gay

Thomas Deutsch has produced a fine book that covers contemporary issues in a comprehensive and fascinating fashion. The format stimulates thought and, one can be certain, discussion. Rather than chapters, the book consists of "cases" that have been cleverly chosen to represent the major therapeutic challenges we all face today. With each case presentation, Dr. Deutsch provides us with a fine summary of the problems and the solutions promulgated by his two or more experts. He has chosen his contributors well and they are all comfortable with their respective points of view. This splendid format provides us with interesting debate and a wealth of information.

Our science continues to progress by "exponential" leaps, while most of us cope best with "linear" progression. Rapid change is bound to bring controversy, as practitioners explore new ways of doing things that a few short years ago could only have been imagined. It is thus appropriate that the editor of this splendid text utilizes the debate format. Such a risky undertaking, however, necessitates a bringing together of the best our specialty has to offer. This task was not easy for our editor, but he has accomplished it in grand fashion. Dr. Deutsch has assembled a stellar group of clinicians and surgeons who describe their approaches to specific problems in patient management. The editor has wisely chosen cases that represent a broad range of clinical problems. The two approaches invariably provide information that is both concise and yet complete. The summary, however, is the strength of the problem-oriented text, for it directs us to the controversy and whets our appetite for the debate and final understanding.

We should "decide all controversies by infallible artillery" but suffice to say, we cannot. The cannoneers are too strong and the battlefield mined with the idiosyncrasies of a multitude of diseases. Dr. Deutsch, however, plays the Greek god and sets in motion the giants of our specialty. Under his careful direction, they grapple with the problems we all face daily in our offices and hospitals. The result, while perhaps frustrating to some who would have but one answer to the most complex of problems, is like a breath of fresh air to those who would think, and work, and move with confidence into the next century. Dr. Deutsch, we who are certain of only one thing, that the future holds change and that our patients will best benefit from fair and honest debate, salute you and your fine chronicle.

J. Terry Ernest, M.D., Ph.D.
Professor and Chairman
Department of Ophthalmology and Visual
* Science*
University of Chicago
Adjunct Professor of Ophthalmology
University of Illinois at Chicago
Chicago, Illinois

PREFACE

Each of us, in the course of everyday practice, is confronted by clinical situations that make us wonder what the "experts" would do. This book is intended to address those questions by providing two different viewpoints to the management of a series of clinical problems.

Because of the unusual format presented in this book, it will be helpful to understand the way in which it was constructed. As the editor, I chose the topics to be covered, wrote the case reports, invited the contributors, and produced the summary that appears with each case. All of these cases are common problems, in most instances derived from my own experience or practice.

Each contributor was invited to write about a specific case and was given some guidelines with respect to the approach I wished him to take. No contributor was given the identity of the other individual responding to that case, nor the guidelines that were given to the other contributor. For purposes of generating a debate, contributors were asked to stick to the guidelines as much as possible. Many of these "debates" were manufactured for the purpose of making interesting reading, and to give the reader more opinions to choose from. Therefore, as would be expected, in some cases the experts disagreed while in others they agreed so thoroughly that there was no actual debate. In each case, however, we do have two approaches.

The inclusion of many authors means that many writing styles, as well as many management approaches, are found in this book. We purposely have not tried to "smooth" the styles by heavily editing the submissions. In most cases you will read the opinions exactly as they arrived, as though you had called the expert on the telephone to solicit advice.

These cases are a potpourri of common ocular problems. It is hoped that these *Ophthalmic Clinical Debates* will be of interest and help to those at all levels of training and practice.

Thomas A. Deutsch, M.D.

ACKNOWLEDGMENTS ___

Editing a book with 51 contributors is a mammoth undertaking. It obviously could not have been accomplished without the assistance and sacrifice of a number of individuals.

David K. Marshall, senior medical editor at Year Book Medical Publishers, had the task of asking me to construct the format for this book, and then talking me into being the editor. He also gave moral support and positive reinforcement as was necessary, expertly guiding this work to publication.

My administrator, secretary, and nursemaid, Judy Linquist, endlessly typed addresses on letters of invitation to prospective contributors, and on notes beseeching them to return their manuscripts.

My wife, Judy, put up with night after night of my own word processing. When I was lazy, she also was available with a gentle reminder that I had work to do.

Finally, the 51 contributors, all busy practitioners, teachers, and researchers, contributed their time and expertise in order to teach us something. Without them, these pages, as well as our understanding of many of the problems faced in this book, would be bare.

I thank them all.

Thomas A. Deutsch, M.D.

CONTENTS _____

SECTION III   GLAUCOMA   101

SECTION *I*————

Cataract Surgery

High Myopia and Implant Power—Four Eyes for the Librarian?

APPROACH 1

Robert M. Sinskey, M.D.

APPROACH 2

Norman S. Jaffe, M.D.

Case 1 _____

High Myopia and Implant Power— Four Eyes for the Librarian?

A 62-year-old librarian has had a progressive decrease in her visual acuity over the past year. Although she has worn a high myopic correction for most of her life, her refraction has changed recently from $-9.00 = 20/20$ (OD), $-10.00 = 20/25$ (OS) to $-11.00 = 20/25$ (OD), $-14.00 = 20/100$ (OS). She has $3+$ nuclear sclerosis in the right eye and $4+$ nuclear sclerosis with $2+$ posterior subcapsular changes in the left eye.

The patient's ophthalmologist has recommended cataract surgery, and she has consented. An intraocular lens calculation has determined the power for emmetropia in the left eye to be 8.0 D. What implant power should be used?

Summary _____

This case presents a common and vexing problem, and it is probable that there is no "right" answer. The patient has been a myope all of her life and is used to wearing glasses. One would assume that she would be perfectly happy to continue being myopic. On the other hand, the patient's ophthalmologist has the opportunity to make her an emmetrope by selecting a low-power implant, a condition that would free her of the need for a distance correction for the first time in nearly 60 years.

In arguing his side, Dr. Sinskey points out that the other eye has also recently become more myopic and may need cataract surgery very soon. If emmetropia is chosen for the first eye, she may soon have the opportunity to be bilaterally emmetropic. It is true that such patients are often so happy that there is a push to remove the second cataract as soon as possible.

Conversely, Dr. Jaffe takes the stance that the patient, having been myopic all of her life and having excellent vision in the second eye at the present time, should be left myopic, though less than in the second eye. He logically takes us through the calculation one can use to determine what implant power to choose depending on the desired amount of residual myopia. The point is made that avoiding the anisometropia that will be inevitable if emmetropia is chosen may also make it possible to avoid premature surgery on the second eye.

Both of these arguments are logical and compelling. The important advice that both discussants offer is to individualize the choice for each patient. It is also our experience that most patients can understand the issues presented in this case and will be of valuable assistance in the decision-making process.

Approach 1 _____

Robert M. Sinskey, M.D.

The history is that of a 62-year-old librarian who has had a progressive decrease in her visual acuity over the past year. Although she has worn a high myopic correction most of her life, her refraction has changed recently from OD −9.00 = 20/20 to −11.00 = 20/25 and OS −10.00 = 20/25 to −14.00 = 20/100. She has a 4+ nuclear sclerosis in the right eye, and in the left eye she has a 4+ nuclear sclerosis with posterior subcapsular changes. The patient's ophthalmologist has recommended cataract surgery and she has consented. The lens power calculation has determined the intraocular lens to be an 8.0 D for emmetropia in the left eye.

The decision to do a cataract extraction in the patient's left eye has been made because of the patient's complaints of visual debility. The options of the residual postoperative refraction have to be explained to the patient, and she has to share in the decision making. The intelligence of the patient also has to be considered. How much the patient can be made to understand about the options has to be taken into account. With the type of patient that I normally see in my practice, it is relatively easy to explain the situation. We show such patients that if we remove the cataract and implant a lens we can eliminate their near sightedness. However, in all likelihood, they will not be able to use the eyes together after surgery, assuming that there was good fusion before surgery. The patient would either have to wear a contact lens postoperatively in the right eye or have a cataract extraction sooner than one normally would if the patient cannot handle anisometropia or a contact lens.

With the degree of nuclear sclerosis this patient has, I have no hesitancy in influencing the patient to enjoy emmetropia or slight myopia in the left eye with the idea that we would probably have to do another cataract extraction with lens implant in the right eye within 3 or 4 months after the first eye has been done. The patients are usually so ecstatic over the results of the first surgery that they push for the surgery in the other eye as soon as possible even though the visual acuity is only reduced to 20/25.

At the time of surgery, I would do a phacoemulsification on this patient and implant a 14.5-mm-overall polypropylene loop using the Sinskey II loop design with a 7-mm optic with no holes and an ultraviolet (UV) filter with 10 degree angulation to the loops. The purpose of the 7-mm optic is not so much for glare control but to act as a barrier to the vitreous coming forward in case a posterior capsulotomy must be performed later on. Obviously, having no holes reduces the possibility of glare and secondary images.

These highly myopic patients clearly need more careful attention to retinal examination. Retinal pre-examination should be done if at all possible and certainly postoperatively. Of course, it is very important to preserve the posterior capsule in these cases at the time of the initial procedure.

Approach 2 _____

Norman S. Jaffe, M.D.

Using a debate format, I will take the position that it would be inadvisable to use an intraocular lens that would make the patient emmetropic postoperatively. Arguments will be presented in favor of residual postoperative myopia, the amount to be discussed.

It is assumed that the patient will undergo an extracapsular cataract extraction or a phacoemulsification for those who would employ it in the presence of 4+ nuclear sclerosis. The question is the power of the posterior chamber lens that should be used in this patient. In making this determination, the past and present life-style of the patient and the status of the opposite eye are crucial.

Life-style

The patient is a librarian who is still active in a profession in which she can remain active for an indeterminate number of years. She has probably had axial myopia since preadolescence and has functioned in a profession that requires good vision. Although not stated in the history, it is assumed that she drives to and from work. She has probably complained of an overall decrease in visual efficiency as a result of an increase in refractive myopia from -10.00 to -14.00 D and a decrease in distance visual acuity from 20/25 to 20/100. These changes have occurred during a period of only 1 year. The complaints are not stated, but it is likely that the patient is disturbed by the resulting anisometropia and the great disparity of visual acuity of the two eyes.

It is assumed that the patient has worn spectacles for nearly a lifetime. If the patient preferred contact lenses, it would have been stated in the history. It is assumed that the patient is not disturbed by using spectacles or, if so, has not successfully used contact lenses in the past. Therefore, it is further assumed that the patient would not object to using spectacles postoperatively.

Opposite Eye

The opposite eye still has good vision with spectacle correction (20/25). It is possible that this might not change significantly for a few years, although it is noted that the myopia has increased from − 9.00 to − 11.00 D during the past year. Therefore, one must be circumspect in planning surgery for the left eye. Using a debate format and for the sake of discussion, I will assume that the patient has tried contact lenses in the past and has been unsuccessful with them or that she does not desire to use them. The surgeon should avoid trying to be a "hero" by making the patient emmetropic in the operated eye if the opposite eye has 11 D of myopia and good corrected visual acuity with little likelihood of contact lens use. This will leave an unhappy patient and might lead to premature surgery for the fellow eye.

Management

I would attempt to restore those conditions that prevailed during the patient's earlier years, i.e., good vision in each eye and spectable correction of the myopia.

We are presented with an intraocular lens (IOL) power calculation of 8.0 D for emmetropia in the eye to have surgery. We are not given the various components of the patient's refraction, but I will assume that the principal cause for her myopia is increased axial length. An important missing piece of information is an IOL power calculation for emmetropia in the opposite eye. It would be important to know whether the patient was always anisometropic because of a significant difference of axial lengths of the two eyes. However, for the sake of discussion it will be assumed that the patient had a similar degree of axial myopia in both eyes. It is important to base the power of the IOL on the axial portion of the myopia and not be influenced by the increase in myopia due to lenticular changes.

It would be helpful to know the patient's refraction before the onset of the cataract. It is likely that this information is available for the type of patient under discussion. Let us assume that her refraction was −8.00 in each eye. A satisfactory method of selecting an IOL power to produce this amount of myopia postoperatively is to employ the old 1.25 rule.[1] It is known that a one-to-one relationship does not exist for each diopter of IOL power change, i.e., a 1 D increase in IOL power does not produce 1 D of residual myopia. Since the residual refractive error is corrected by a spectacle lens worn at a vertex distance of about 12 mm, a change in lens power within the eye has a slightly different effectivity. The 1.25 rule states that for each diopter of IOL change only 0.8 D change in the residual refraction results. Thus, if the patient requires an 8.00 D lens for emmetropia, an 18.00 D posterior chamber lens should produce a postoperative myopia of −8.00 D. This is arrived at by multiplying 8 × 1.25, or 10.00 D. The latter is added to the 8.00 D lens required to produce emmetropia. Examples of this are shown in the following table.

For the patient under discussion, the 1.25 rule is used as follows:

TABLE 1–1.

Residual Myopia vs. IOL Power; 8.0 D for Emmetropia

Residual Myopia	IOL Power (D)
Plano	8.00
−1.00	9.25
−2.00	10.50
−3.00	11.75
−4.00	13.00
−5.00	14.25
−6.00	15.50
−7.00	16.75
−8.00	18.00

I would use an 18.00 D posterior chamber lens for this patient. This would leave about − 8.00 D of residual myopia. The patient should be reasonably comfortable with the postoperative anisometropia (the unoperated eye has a − 11.00 D refraction). If the opposite eye develops an operable cataract, an appropriate IOL power can be chosen to conform with the first eye. I would aim at 2 D less residual myopia, although this is optional.

Disadvantages of This Approach

Most patients would prefer to be emmetropic in both eyes postoperatively. If the patient were able to tolerate a contact lens in the unoperated eye, the operated eye could be made approximately emmetropic. A trial of contact lens wear can be undertaken before surgery in order to make this determination. The fellow eye will probably become more myopic due to lenticular changes while still retaining relatively good corrected visual acuity. If the patient were able to manage a contact lens in this eye, a simple change in lens power could be made to adjust to the change in myopia.

In conclusion, there are several approaches to this problem. Management should be determined by the past and present lifestyle of the patient and the condition of the opposite eye.

Reference

1. Jaffe NS: *Cataract Surgery and Its Complications,* ed 4. St Louis, CV Mosby Co, 1984, pp 145–146.

Pseudophakic Cystoid Macular Edema—Do Lenses Cause Leaks?

APPROACH 1

Manus C. Kraff, M.D.

APPROACH 2

David H. Orth, M.D.

Case 2 _____

Pseudophakic Cystoid Macular Edema—Do Lenses Cause Leaks?

A 75-year-old man had cataract surgery 6 weeks ago. At the time of surgery, a tear was made inadvertently in the central posterior capsule, but vitreous was not encountered, and a posterior chamber implant was placed in the capsular bag. At the 3-week examination, the best corrected visual acuity was 20/25, and there was mild anterior chamber reaction. Today, the best corrected visual acuity is 20/50, mild anterior-chamber reaction is still present, and there is mild cystoid macular edema (CME) seen with the contact lens.

The patient would like to know whether the implant has caused the edema and whether any therapy is necessary.

Summary

The revolution in cataract surgery has continued to result in changes in technique. In most cases, a skilled surgeon can implant a posterior chamber intraocular lens (PC-IOL) even if a small- to moderate-sized opening appears in the posterior capsule. This case presents such a situation in which CME has developed. It is discussed from the standpoints of a busy cataract surgeon and an experienced retinal specialist.

Dr. Kraff stresses the importance of decision making at the time of surgery. Surgeons must not only assess the damage but also realistically evaluate their various skills in dealing with the problem. It is essential to inspect the capsular ring in order to determine whether sufficient capsule is present to support a posterior chamber lens.

Management of CME is covered by Dr. Orth. Although periocular and topical steroids or systemic antiprostaglandin (anti-PG) agents are recommended, many of the patients will respond initially, but the vision will deteriorate when treatment with the medications is withdrawn. Eyes in which there is vitreous incarcerated in the wound should be considered for vitrectomy.

Both of the authors stress the importance of proper management of the vitreous prior to implantation of any lens. In the past few years, vitreous cleanup after rupture of the posterior capsule has become easier because of the availability of automated equipment. Every cataract surgeon must become proficient in the careful removal of vitreous and know the circumstances in which it is appropriate to implant either an anterior or a posterior chamber lens or no lens at all.

Approach 1 _____

Manus C. Kraff, M.D.

What is the proper surgical and postoperative management of a patient when capsular rupture occurs (Fig 2–1)? In some cases, peripheral ruptures are not detected immediately, especially if the surgeon is less experienced. If such a rupture is not detected and a PC-IOL is placed in the capsule without bridging the rupture such that the lens and haptics are put in a support area, the patient may subsequently experience the sunrise or sunset syndrome associated with subluxation of the lens. Even without subluxation, a patient with capsular rupture, especially with vitreous manipulation, may develop CME, as in the case described. Not only will the CME need to be treated properly, but the primary cause of these events will need to be determined, both for proper management of the case and in order to answer the patient's questions concerning the cause of the problem: was the CME caused by the cataract surgery itself or by the insertion of the PC-IOL (i.e., should the lens have been inserted)? In this particular case, it was probably the cataract surgery and concurrent capsular rupture that caused the edema rather than the implant itself.

If capsular rupture is recognized at the time of surgery, as it was in this case, it is necessary to assess both the location and the extent of the rupture because these parameters will determine the proper surgical management of the case. If there is adequate peripheral support, that is, if the lens and haptics can be placed in a support area, then the surgeon may proceed to insert the PC-IOL in the ciliary sulcus anterior to the capsular bag while bridging the gap and taking care to properly control the vitreous by using air or a viscoelastic substance. The ciliary sulcus is preferred over bag fixation because of the increased support in this case. If vit-

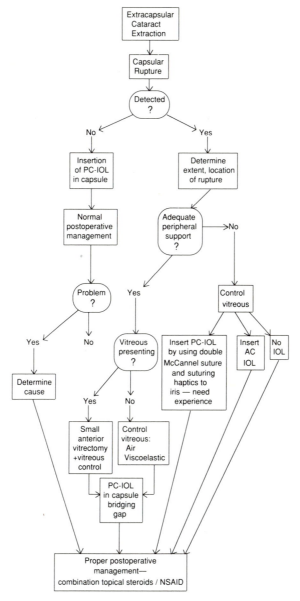

FIG 2–1.
Algorithm for proper surgical and postoperative management of capsular rupture.

reous is encountered, the surgeon should first perform a small anterior vitrectomy using an automated system and then reinspect the peripheral support; if adequate, the IOL may be inserted and the gap bridged.

If the rupture is too large and there is no adequate peripheral support for the insertion of the PC-IOL in the capsular bag, three options remain available. Obviously, the surgeon may decide against insertion of an IOL. I believe that a lens *should* be implanted if at all possible. Adequate evaluation of the extent of the rupture and/or vitreous presentation should make this possible in all but the most extreme cases. If it isn't possible, later secondary implantation or epikeratophakia are alternatives if a contact lens fails.

A second option, then, is to insert an anterior-chamber IOL (AC-IOL). There is really no question that in uneventful cases the implantation of a PC-IOL is preferable to the use of an anterior-chamber one. Furthermore, if the rupture were not too large, as in the case described, I would have put in the PC-IOL, as the surgeon did. However, the one-piece polymethylmethacrylate (PMMA), flexible-design, anterior-chamber lenses currently in use appear to be quite safe and useful in a situation where insufficient capsular support is available for posterior-chamber lens implantation.

Still another option in the face of a large capsular rupture with little zonular support is to insert a PC-IOL by using a double McCannel suture and suturing the haptics to the iris. This solution should be considered only by the experienced surgeon, duly considering the status of the eye. This option, to me, is less desirable than an anterior chamber lens, given the level of technical surgical expertise required with this former approach.

Postoperative management of cases with capsular rupture is also important. I prefer to attempt to prevent CME prophylactically by using a combination of topical steroids and nonsteroidal anti-inflammatory drugs (NSAID). I recommend flurbiprofen (Ocufen) drops, beginning four times daily, with a decreasing dosage over a 6-month period. Flurbiprofen is currently Food and Drug Administration (FDA) approved, though not for this indication.

Approach 2 _____

David H. Orth, M.D.

The history is that of a 75-year-old man who had cataract surgery 6 weeks ago. At the time of surgery, a tear was inadvertently made in the center of the posterior capsule. However, there was no vitreous encountered, and a posterior-chamber implant was placed in the capsular bag. Three weeks after surgery, the best corrected visual acuity was 20/25. There was a mild anterior-chamber reaction at that time. At this most recent examination, the best corrected visual acuity was 20/50. There is still a mild anterior-chamber reaction, and with contact lens examination, there is evidence of mild CME.

Several issues arise from this history and sequence of events:

1. The patient would like to know whether the IOL is the cause for the CME. He is told that the CME is related primarily to the fact that he has undergone intraocular surgery and is not necessarily related to the implantation of the posterior chamber lens. He is told that prior to the era of lens implantation CME was the most frequent visually disabling complication of cataract surgery. In the immediate postoperative period, it occurred in as many as 60% to 77% of the patients who had undergone the routine type of intracapsular cataract extraction without the implantation of an IOL. In fact, there have been studies that suggest that a planned extracapsular cataract extraction with lens implantation may lower the incidence of CME.

It is also pointed out to the patient that there may be other causes that increase the possibility of CME developing. These include the fact that the frequency of CME increases with age and also increases in those patients who may have diabetes mellitus and/or systemic hypertension.

2. Is the IOL implantation appropriate when there has been capsular rupture with or without vitreous manipulation? There is no contraindication to the implantation of a posterior chamber lens in cases where there has been an inadvertent capsular rupture and no involvement of the vitreous gel. In fact, many of the early cases of extracapsular cataract surgery with posterior-chamber lens implantation consisted of doing a primary central capsulotomy during the initial operative procedure.

In cases where there has been vitreous herniation or vitreous loss during the primary procedure, I would recommend that the idea of implanting a posterior-chamber lens should probably be aborted. With the improved vitrectomy instruments that are now available, an uncomplicated anterior vitrectomy can easily be done, and an anterior chamber lens can be implanted. It is imperative that all of the vitreous be removed from the anterior chamber and the surgeon make sure that there is no vitreous incarcerated in the cataract wound since this may lead to long-standing irreversible CME.

3. When should treatment be initiated for CME, and what are the various forms of management? The management of CME is directed toward the premise that this postoperative complication is secondary to a low-grade intraocular inflammation. Therefore, the use of topical, periocular, and systemic corticosteroids as well as inhibitors of PG synthesis should be considered in the management of CME. This treatment could either be prophylactic (preoperative) or therapeutic (postoperative).

When a patient reports that initially, after cataract surgery with lens implantation, the vision was good and over a period of weeks to months became blurred, a high index of suspicion should arise that CME has developed. It is important that the CME be documented by fluorescein angiography. The extent of the edema will frequently determine the prognosis for vision if the edema can be reduced. If the patient has a large central confluent cyst or there is foveal damage, it is unlikely that he will regain an improvement in the visual acuity, even if a therapeutic agent reduces the amount of edema. Therefore, early detection and treatment are desirable.

The longer the edema is present, the greater the chances of developing a confluent cyst and having secondary irreversible changes within the sensory retina.

Management with corticosteroids can be topical, periocular, or systemic. In general, topical corticosteroids have been thought to be ineffective in the therapy for CME. In some cases where the patients have been steroid responders and there has been an increase in the intraocular pressure, there has also been a subsequent decrease in the amount of CME. There have also been studies indicating the potential benefit of both systemic and periocular corticosteroids in reducing CME and improving vision. However, in most of these cases, recurrences were common once the effect of the corticosteroids was diminished. Since some of these reports have been promising, a well-designed randomized prospective clinical trial would be worthwhile.

Anti-PGs or PG synthesis inhibitors also have shown some promise in reducing clinically evident CME. PGs have been found to be mediators of inflammation in the eye. These unsaturated fatty acids are synthesized in the eye in response to a wide variety of traumatic stimuli such as mechanical stroking of the iris. There have been only a few studies that have used PG synthesis inhibitors for the treatment of CME. None of the reports have been convincing that systemic PG synthesis inhibitors such as indomethacin are of any value in decreasing the presence of established CME. There has been one study using topical PG synthesis inhibitors for CME. Although this double-masked randomized trial showed no statistically significant effect, there were several patients who did have an improvement, and recurrences occurred once treatment with the drops was discontinued. Most of the work reported in the literature, to this point in time, has been in studying the value of topical PG synthesis inhibitors for prophylaxis of CME.

As far as the surgical management of CME is concerned, this would fall into the possibility of photocoagulation or vitrectomy surgery. In the late 1960s and 1970s, several investigators attempted to seal the perifoveal leaking capillaries in the macula that were demonstrated on angiography. None of these studies showed a positive result to laser treatment. This would certainly be expected since the actual cause of the edema, i.e., low-grade inflammation and possible PG synthesis, have not been addressed. As far as vitrectomy surgery is concerned, if there is a lot of vitreous gel in the anterior chamber as well as incarcerated in the cataract wound, this should be removed by using one of the new-generation vitrectomy instruments. In my opinion, there is no longer a place for employing cellulose sponges and scissors in order to remove vitreous in the anterior segment of the eye.

Recommendations for Treatment

When a patient presents with a history of reduced vision and decreased visual acuity has been documented, fluorescein angiography is done to document the extent and type of CME that is present. Treatment is instituted immediately. I try to avoid systemic corticosteroid therapy since many of these patients are elderly and because of the potential serious systemic complications. If the patient is not a steroid responder to topical medication, I will consider the use of 60 mg of prednisone as a sub-Tenon's injection. This will be combined with topical corticosteroid drops three times a day. In those cases where periocular corticosteroids are not used, I will recommend systemic anti-PG medication such as fenoprofen calcium (Nalfon) if there are no systemic contraindications. The patients are advised as to the side effects of Nalfon and are told to discontinue treatment with the drug if any of the side effects arise. The usual dose is 300 to 600 mg three times a day for 3 weeks to see whether there is any response in reducing the CME and improving the vision.

References

1. Federman JL, Annesley WH Jr, Sarin LK, et al: Vitrectomy and cystoid macular edema. *Ophthalmology* 1980; 87:622–628.
2. Fung WE: Anterior vitrectomy for chronic aphakic cystoid macular edema. *Ophthalmology* 1980; 87:189–193.
3. Klein RM, Katzin HM, Yannuzzi LA: The effect of indomethacin pretreatment on aphakic cystoid macular edema. *Am J Ophthalmol* 1979; 87:487–489.

4. Kraff MC, Sanders DR, Jampol LM, et al: Prophylaxis of pseudo-phakic cystoid macular edema with topical Indomethacin. *Ophthalmology* 1982; 89:885–890.
5. Miyake K: Prevention of cystoid macular edema after lens extraction by topical indomethacin (1). A preliminary report. *Graefes Arch Klin Exp Ophthalmol* 1977; 203:81–88.
6. Miyake K: Prevention of cystoid macular edema after lens extraction by topical indomethacin. II. A control study in bilateral extraction. *Jpn J Ophthalmol* 1978; 22:80–94.
7. Meredith TA, Kenyon KR, Singerman LJ, et al: Perifoveal vascular leakage and macular edema after intracapsular cataract extraction. *Br J Ophthalmol* 1976; 60:765–769.
8. Orth DH, Henry MD: Management of Irvine-Gass syndrome using pars plana vitrectomy, in Emery JM (ed): *Current Concepts in Cataract Surgery. Selected Proceedings of the Fifth Biennial Cataract Surgical Congress.* St Louis, CV Mosby Co, 1978, pp 375–380.
9. Stern AL, Taylor DM, Dalburg LA, et al: Pseudophakic cystoid maculopathy: A study of 50 cases. *Ophthalmology* 1981; 88:942–946.
10. Yannuzzi LA, Klein RM, Wallyn RH, et al: Ineffectiveness of indomethacin in the treatment of chronic cystoid macular edema. *Am J Ophthalmol* 1977; 84:517–519.
11. Zweng HC, Little HL, Peabody RR: Laser photocoagulation of macular lesions. *Trans Am Acad Ophthalmol Otolaryngol* 1968; 72:377–388.

Nd:YAG Posterior Capsulotomy—Who and When?

APPROACH 1

Robert C. Drews, M.D.

APPROACH 2

Carmen A. Puliafito, M.D.

Case 3 _____

Nd:YAG Posterior Capsulotomy— Who and When?

A 58-year-old woman had cataract surgery with an implant 3 months ago. At the 6-week examination, the best corrected visual acuity was 20/20. The patient notes that the acuity has slowly worsened, and refraction now indicates a best corrected visual acuity of 20/80. The eye is quiet, and the posterior capsule is hazy. A 20/80 view of the retina reveals a normal disc and macula.

The patient wants to know whether her vision can be improved with the Nd:YAG laser. How can one predict whether the visual acuity will improve with laser treatment, and what is the best timing for the treatment?

Summary _____

This case brings up the common problem of the patient with vision that begins to diminish in the relatively early post–cataract extraction period. The surgeon is faced with the task of determining whether the visual loss is due to opacification of the posterior capsule and then advising the patient as to the chances of improvement after a laser posterior capsulotomy.

Retinal causes of reduced vision should be ruled out, and Dr. Drews stresses the importance of retinal consultation if there is any suspicion of retinal pathology. He favors the potential acuity meter (PAM) as a means of predicting for the patient what the potential gain in visual acuity might be.

Dr. Puliafito notes the importance of the direct ophthalmoscopic view of the retina in the evaluation of the degree of capsular opacification. The slit-lamp appearance, the view with the indirect ophthalmoscope, and the results of glare testing can all mislead the surgeon either toward or away from implicating the posterior capsule as the cause of reduced vision.

The single most important test that is performed prior to posterior capsulotomy is refraction. It is extremely common for the refractive error to continue changing for at least a year after cataract surgery, and a simple test of the visual acuity with the present glasses is insufficient evidence of a reduction in vision.

Approach 1 _____

Robert C. Drews, M.D.

A 58-year-old patient has come in wanting a YAG laser posterior capsulotomy 3 months after cataract surgery with lens implantation. She had 20/20 vision 6 weeks after surgery, and the vision has now fallen to 20/80. Ophthalmoscopically the decreased vision seems to be accounted for by haze of the posterior lens capsule.

Other Possible Causes of Early Decreased Visual Acuity

It is very uncommon for a posterior lens capsule to cloud so quickly after cataract surgery. It may be cloudy at once, of course. But for the patient to have 20/20 vision 6 weeks after surgery and 20/80 vision another 6 weeks later is highly unusual. For this reason other possible causes of the decreased visual acuity need to be ruled out *before* a YAG capsulotomy is performed. Otherwise these causes of the decreased vision may be blamed on the YAG capsulotomy and the surgeon who performs the procedure.

The patient may already have cystoid macular edema (CME). If the haze of the posterior lens capsule prevents an adequate view, referral to a retinal specialist is indicated, and fluorescein angiography may be necessary to confirm or deny this possibility.

Even if macular edema is found, however, the possibility that this patient may have a retinal detachment must be seriously considered and ruled out. It is easy to miss a detachment, especially if it is inferior or relatively flat. A visual field can be very helpful. Indirect ophthalmoscopy is essential, and referral to a retinal specialist should be made if there is any doubt.

Differential diagnosis should include ischemic optic neuropathy or so-called postoperative optic neuritis. A visual field may be helpful, again.

Other extremely rare conditions have to include such things as occult peripheral malignant melanoma missed preoperatively because of the patient's cataract. By now the reader may gather that I would probably refer this patient to a retinal surgeon in consultation if I had any doubt that the decreased vision was due to a condition other than clouding of the lens capsule.

Microhyphema can occur anytime after surgery but presents an episodic rather than a steady downhill course. Examination of the corneal endothelium typically shows a pseudo-Krukenberg's spindle of red blood cells in a fan-shaped pattern inferiorly. While looking with the slit lamp, be sure the haze seen ophthalmoscopically is due to the posterior lens capsule and not to microcystic edema of the corneal epithelium (from increased intraocular pressure) or the cornea generally (from endothelial decompensation).

The protocol says nothing about anterior-chamber reaction or vitritis, but if this eye is not quiet, one has to consider the possibility of a smoldering endophthalmitis from such organisms as *Staphylococcus epidermidis* or *Propionobacterium acnes.*

Rapid Clouding of Posterior Lens Capsule

Rapid clouding of the posterior lens capsule is unusual. It is most frequently seen when there are large amounts of cortical material left at the end of surgery either because these were unrecognized or because some intraoperative event such as positive vitreous pressure or rupture of the capsule or zonule prevented a thorough cleanout. Such material can proliferate across the posterior lens capsule either in the form of fibrosis (fibrous metaplasia) or as epithelial pearls. It would be unusual to have epithelial pearls proliferate across the posterior lens capsule this rapidly, but I suppose anything is possible. If the decreased vision is due to cortical material rather than fibrosis, this would be better aspirated without opening the posterior capsule so early after surgery.

The protocol does not say what type of intraocular lens was

used, but it is reported that silicone lenses can be associated with rapid fibrosis of the posterior lens capsule.

A recently cited cause of clouding of the posterior lens capsule is the presence of a low-grade endophthalmitis within the capsular sac due to *P acnes*. If cortical or endocapsular material is aspirated, it should be cultured anaerobically and part of the aspirate examined with a Gram stain.

The time course is much too rapid, again, but unusual membrane formation should also include the differential diagnosis of the possibility of epithelial downgrowth. This possibility must be especially considered whenever a membrane reforms rapidly after a capsulotomy has been performed (either with a YAG laser or with a knife).

Testing Visual Potential

It is surprising how many patients I see in consultation for visual problems who can be helped with a good manifest refraction. Refraction of the postoperative patient can be greatly assisted by making a keratometer measurement and using the cylinder and axis found as a starting point in the refraction.

The lowly pinhole gives useful information in over 80% of the patients that I try it on. It is simple, quick, and easy, and when it produces a dramatic increase in vision, the patient and relatives (and doctor) are so impressed with the test results that they forget any possible disappointment in the simplicity of the test itself.

When the pinhole does not avail, more sophisticated instrumentation can be employed. There is a difference of opinion as to whether laser fringes or the potential acuity meter (PAM) is more useful. Either one has been reported to give false-positive results in the face of CME. I personally prefer the PAM.

The purpose of these tests, again, is to avoid unattainable expectations with subsequent disappointment after the capsulotomy. In the absence of observable retinal problems—and in the presence of *significant* clouding of the posterior lens capsule—I will almost always do a YAG posterior capsulotomy anyway to eliminate at least that part of the problem caused by the clouding of the posterior capsule and to gain a better view of the fundus.

When to Do a YAG Laser Posterior Capsulotomy

Although many papers given at meetings have cited an almost zero incidence of CME if (surgical) posterior capsulotomy is deferred a year after surgery, few ophthalmologists today will wait that long if (1) there is significant clouding of the posterior lens capsule and (2) the eye has become completely quiet. To do a capsulotomy on an inflamed eye invites (or perhaps will disclose) CME.

The Capsulotomy Itself

It seems that, with all laser work, the frequency and severity of complications is proportional to the amount of energy poured into the eye. This is true not only for the YAG laser but also for argon, xenon, etc. (Maybe this is true for surgery too!?) Accordingly, one of the early principles laid down by Danielle Aron-Rosa was the use of minimal energy to perform the capsulotomy. It is not unusual to see her perform a capsulotomy in one to three pulses. I started out by making a circular opening using 30 to 60 pulses (and sometimes worrying about the operculum), but these days I tend to make a linear or slightly cruciate incision with 3 to 10 pulses. These usually open up quite nicely and are more than adequate.

Likewise, I used to always dilate the pupil, but now I find that I can work quite well through the normal-sized pupil, with better centering of the capsulotomy. It is helpful to have the patient look slight eccentrically to avoid reflections. If gaze is diverted first slightly to one side and then the other, the capsulotomy can be enlarged beyond the edge of the pupil quite nicely.

Unless a large capsulotomy is needed for retinal work (such as panretinal photocoagulation), a capsulotomy 2 mm in diameter is usually quite sufficient. Occasionally a young patient is disturbed by glare from the edges of the opaque capsule in a relatively large pupil at night.

Care After Laser Treatment

Any capsulotomy, whether performed by a laser or a knife, may lead to increased intraocular pressure, uveitis, CME, or retinal detachment. The evaluations performed on the patient before laser treatment should be repeated afterward, and the patient will usually need follow-up examination as well. The Food and Drug Administration (FDA) has reported that the incidence of retinal detachment after capsulotomy is about 1%. Interestingly, this is a complication that is omitted from the standard FDA informed consent form for YAG laser posterior capsulotomy!

Conclusion

Although I would prefer to wait a little longer postoperatively, after a thorough and favorable workup I would have no objection to having this patient receive the capsulotomy for which she is so anxious. Because the case is unusual, I would just worry more—and be sure that my records are complete, that appropriate informed consent has been obtained, and that my discussions with the patient and her relatives are well documented.

Approach 2 _____

Carmen A. Puliafito, M.D.

Postoperative opacification of initially clear posterior capsules occurs frequently in patients after extracapsular cataract extraction of senile cataracts. In large series of extracapsular cataract extractions, up to 50% of patients eventually require capsulotomy. It may be difficult to judge the contribution of the patient's capsular opacity to the patient's overall visual deficit in some cases. Nevertheless, clinical experience and the results of several published investigations provide guidelines to the proper evaluation of posterior capsule opacification. It goes without saying that every patient requires a complete ophthalmic history and examination before capsulotomy, including notation of medical history, topical and systemic medications, vision, intraocular pressure in both eyes, slit-lamp examination, fundus examination, and refraction. Although the risks of posterior capsulotomy are small, serious sight-threatening complications can occur, and this procedure should not be performed without due consideration. Written informed consent should always be obtained.

The History

In cases where the examination is equivocal, the history may be of decisive importance. Patients in whom postoperative visual acuity has never been good require very careful evaluation prior to capsulotomy. In my experience, many of these patients have some cause for decreased vision other than or in addition to capsular opacification, in particular, macular dysfunction (i.e., CME, age-related maculopathy, or diabetic macular edema). Moreover, if the history reveals that the initial cataract surgery was complicated by vitreous loss or capsular rupture, a high index of suspicion for CME should be the rule. Such cases merit particularly careful preoperative evaluation; fluorescein angiography should be performed if macular pathology is suspected. Similar care is justified in cases where the patient has a known antecedent retinal or macular disorder. Conversely, if the patient has had excellent vision postoperatively and presents with decreased vision, glare, or another disturbance of vision attributable to capsular changes, capsulotomy usually produces a gratifying result.

Slit-Lamp Examination

Slit-lamp evaluation is an essential part of the evaluation before posterior capsulotomy, but the limits of this examination technique are all too infrequently stressed, particularly since many clinicians make the decision to perform a capsulotomy solely on the basis of biomicroscopic evaluation. When vision is decreased because of severe capsular fibrosis or by extensive, dense Elschnig's epithelial pearl formation, slit-lamp examination is usually satisfactory. However, it must be remembered that some capsular opacities that are impressive in oblique slit-lamp illumination may be insignificant against the red reflex. These opacities may cause little visual difficulty.

Direct Ophthalmoscopy/Retinoscopy

Perhaps the single most reliable technique for assessing capsular opacity is direct ophthalmoscopy since visibility of retinal details correlates with the patient's view of the world. Retinoscopy and the red reflex seen at the slit lamp or with direct or indirect ophthalmoscopy may also reveal significant optical disturbances. The fundus view using the 90-D lens, Hruby lens, or Goldmann lens may also allow accurate assessment of capsular clouding, whereas the indirect ophthalmoscope can penetrate significant capsular opacities and thus may be misleading.

Retinal Examination/Fluorescein Angiography

All patients undergoing capsulotomy should have a careful macular examination since this is the most common reason for failure of capsulotomy to improve vision. Examination of the retinal periphery is recommended for patients with high myopia, a history of lattice retinal degeneration, or a history of retinal detachment since there is some evidence that such patients are at higher risk for developing the complication of retinal detachment following capsulotomy.

Mild CME can be difficult to detect even by careful biomicroscopic examination, and therefore fluorescein angiography should be performed in cases where CME is suspected. CME is a relative but not absolute contraindication to capsulotomy. There has been a concern that capsulotomy in the presence of CME might increase the severity of the macular edema. However, there are cases in which both capsular opacification and macular edema each play a role in decreasing acuity. The author has performed capsulotomies in three such patients with angiographically demonstrated macular edema and significant capsular opacification. In these cases, vision improved substantially, and the macular edema did not worsen either angiographically or clinically. In such cases, I recommend 4 to 8 weeks of systemic and topical therapy with a nonsteroidal anti-inflammatory agent prior to capsulotomy in attempt to decrease CME prior to proceeding with capsulotomy.

Glare Testing/Contrast Sensitivity

Preoperative glare testing such as with the Miller-Nadler glare tester adds little to the preoperative evaluation of patients with posterior capsular opacification. In the one report that studied this issue, it was found that glare and visual acuity were correlated preoperatively and usually improved concomitantly. The only situation in which glare testing may be useful is when a patient has significant subjective complaints (e.g., glare during night driving) associated with relatively good visual acuity (for instance, 20/25 to 20/30) and a clear posterior capsule with linear wrinkling. Contrast sensitivity testing does not have a role in routine preoperative evaluation of patients undergoing capsulotomy.

Laser or White Light Interferometry/Potential Acuity Meter

Laser or white light interferometry (LI) and the PAM have very limited value in the preoperative evaluation of patients undergoing capsulotomy, primarily because of an unacceptably high false-negative rate (i.e., those cases in which no improvement was predicted but improvement actually occurred) that has been documented in three clinical studies. Page found a false-negative rate of 23.7% in a series of 140 cases evaluated with the Rodenstock LI; Klein found a false-negative rate of 42% with an LI and 33% with the PAM. A high false-negative rate was also noted in the study by Belcher and coworkers. Diffuse posterior capsular opacification that precludes the delivery of light through a clear portion of the capsule was the most likely cause of the high false-negative rates noted. In contrast, a positive result on either test has been shown to have a good predictive value. Even this finding, however, needs to be qualified since both PAM and LI tend to give false-positive readings in the presence of CME. In summary, the use of PAM or LI adds little to the preoperative assessment made by careful clinical examination combined with the selective use of fluorescein angiography.

Timing of Capsulotomy

Retinal complications (i.e., retinal detachment and CME) are rare, and there is no evidence that capsulotomy as soon as 4 weeks following surgery increases this rate of complication. In the era of invasive surgical capsulotomy, it was sometimes stated that capsulotomy should be delayed until at least 6 months following initial surgery since this reduces the rate of CME. This has not been the case with Nd:YAG laser capsulotomy. Capsulotomy, if indicated, can be performed as soon as postsurgical inflammation has subsided.

Bibliography

1. Klein TB, Slomovic AR, Parrish RK II, et al: Visual acuity prediction before neodymium-YAG laser posterior capsulotomy. *Ophthalmology* 1986; 93:808–810.
2. Lang TA, Lindstrom RL: Efficacy of laser interferometry in predicting visual result of YAG laser posterior capsulotomy. *J Am Intraocul Implant Soc* 1985; 11:367–371.
3. Spurny RC, Zaldivar R, Belcher CD III, et al: Instruments for predicting visual acuity. A clinical comparison. *Arch Ophthalmol* 1986; 104:196–200.
4. Steinert RF, Puliafito CA: *The Nd-YAG Laser in Ophthalmology: Principles and Clinical Applications of Photodisruption.* Philadelphia, WB Saunders Co, 1985.

Postoperative Astigmatism—Where to Cut?

APPROACH 1

Richard C. Troutman, M.D.

APPROACH 2

Jonathan B. Rubenstein, M.D.

Postoperative Astigmatism—Where To Cut?

A 68-year-old man who had cataract surgery 3 months ago now has a refraction of $-3.00 + 5.00 \times 180 = 20/25$. There appears to be a slight wound gape. The other eye, which is phakic, has a refraction of $-1.00 = 20/20$.

What is the best way to correct this unwanted against-the-rule astigmatism?

Summary

Modern cataract surgery has progressed to a point where the predictability of the outcome is the highest ever. However, occasionally there is a surprise, as in the case of this patient where a large amount of against-the-rule astigmatism has developed 3 months after surgery.

Dr. Troutman discusses the importance of suturing technique in the avoidance and treatment of this astigmatism. The use of a block resection of the cornea at the margin of the wound is often necessary to correct against-the-rule astigmatism with the magnitude found in this patient.

The use of incisional refractive surgical techniques is discussed by Dr. Rubenstein. He advocates the use of transverse incisions (T-cuts) in cases where the spherical equivalent is nearly plano and the addition of semiradial cuts where there is myopic astigmatism. Relaxing incisions can also be useful.

Both of these astigmatism experts emphasize the importance of preoperative evaluation and intraoperative control of the astigmatism. It is also possible to manipulate the postoperative cylinder amount and axis through educated placement of the cataract incision and sutures.

Approach 1

Richard C. Troutman, M.D.

The treatment of this 68-year-old patient's eye will vary according to his preoperative and postoperative history.

Assuming an intraocular lens has been placed, an A-scan must have been done prior to surgery. Preoperative keratometry measurements could show the astigmatism to be pre-existing. In such a case, if the primary incision was intracorneal, a Troutman wedge or block resection at the incisional area to steepen the flatter vertical meridian is indicated. Multiple interrupted elastic monofilament sutures are placed and tightened under surgical keratometry control to induce an overcorrection of approximately 3 D. The suture loops are left in place for no less than 3 months. They are then removed sequentially until sphericity is approached. If two or more sutures still remain, these are left indefinitely and removed only if they surface or degrade and become irritating.

If the incision was made in or posterior to the corneal scleral sulcus, it will be stepped or oblique, and including it in a block or wedge excision is difficult. Here the wedge or block is removed anterior to the primary incision by making the posterior cut of the block excision to approximately three fourths of the scleral depth. The excision is delimited anteriorly, about 0.75 mm wide, and freed at its base in the corneal scleral junction. Care should be taken not to penetrate the anterior chamber to avoid incarceration of iris, capsule, or vitreous. The closing interrupted suture loops require slightly less tension for apposition than required in a corneal excision. About 3 D of overcorrection should be induced. These subconjunctival sutures are left in place indefinitely unless after 3 months by photokeratometry one or several appear to be inducing an astigmatic band. Offending sutures may be released by cutting at the anterior loop as it enters the cornea and allowed to retract under the conjunctiva. The cut loop need not be removed unless it projects through the conjunctiva. The surgeon is cautioned never to remove tight suture loops until the early overcorrection decreases and becomes stabilized.

Should the corneal curvature have been spherical preoperatively, symmetrical to the other cornea, postoperative against-the-rule astigmatism almost always indicates an internal or external wound gape or dehiscence. Was this condition present immediately after surgery, or did it develop since the last postoperative visit? In the former case a faulty wound closure is the cause and must be resutured at once. In the latter case it is likely caused by a trauma that has loosened or broken a suture or sutures. It is unlikely that a monofilament nylon interrupted or continuous suture that has already been verified as firmly tied at surgery would loosen spontaneously. If multiple interrupted sutures were used, the wound should be sufficiently protected so as not to release a broad-enough sector to induce 5 D of astigmatism. With continuous sutures wound separation can occur only if not protected by interrupted stay sutures.

If repair of an immediate dehiscence has been delayed, some fibroblastic proliferation will extend across the wound. This could be accompanied by incarceration of iris, lens material, or vitreous in the posterior wound. The latter should be ruled out by a gonioscopic examination of the internal wound. If clear, it may be found to be gaping. Following trauma a deeply sutured wound usually will only gape anteriorly. However, if the wound was sutured only in its anterior one half to one third, then the dehiscence is posterior and usually extends through and through. The conjunctiva is dissected from over a corneoscleral wound, and the external wound is examined directly. Loosened suture loops can be seen and replaced. If there has been an attempt at fibroblastic repair, then it is necessary to do a block excision of the fibroblastic material to freshen wound edges before suturing. A slight overcorrection, about 3 D, should be verified by the surgical keratometer. I have not seen such a through-and-through dehiscence in deeply sutured corneal incisions, but it could occur from several sutures being loosened in a sector. With through-and-through sutures in place the posterior wound remains closed, and all that is necessary is to remove any loosened suture loops and replace them.

A significant trauma can break any wound, and it is essential to debride the wound of iris, lens capsule, or vitreous that may be incarcerated. Sodium hyaluronate (Healon) injected into the anterior chamber at the site will tamponade the iris to facilitate suturing.

Did the patient have, from the time of surgery, no complications and a normal-curvature cornea and then present with pain, a shallow anterior chamber, and a wound dehiscence *without* history of trauma? Here suture release is probably related to increased intraocular pressure from a pupillary block. If the block can be relieved medically or by laser iridectomy, the astigmatism will decrease as the elastic monofilament sutures spring the wound back in position. In shallowly sutured incisions such flattening can persist without apparent external wound dehiscence. Gonioscopy of the internal incision for gaping and incarceration should be performed. If present, when intraocular pressure is normalized, a full-thickness resuturing of the wound should be performed. The surgical keratometer should be used to verify a moderate overcorrection, 2 to 3 D, from the suture compression at the end of the procedure. This will decay toward sphericity. If it does not, selective suture removal is performed according to photokeratoscopic findings.

The final and least likely cause of wound-induced corneal flattening is inaccurate vertical wound alignment. A series of short, shallow suture bites in the scleral lip of the wound with correspondingly deeper bites into the cornea lip will elevate the corneal wound edge above the scleral wound to induce flattening of the wound meridian. Because of poor healing, when sutures are released, such a wound closure results in a severe against-the-rule astigmatism. In this instance a block resection is necessary. The defective incisional area must be excised and the new wound edges exactly aligned and closed with interrupted sutures.

The postoperative care of these patients is important since the multiple surgeries may cause delayed corneal problems. Again, there may be persistent increased intraocular pressure because of peripheral synechiae resulting from loss of the chamber at the time of the dehiscence. This may have been unobserved by the surgeon. A sequential evaluation of intraocular pressure and gonioscopy as compared with a normal fellow eye when possible will confirm that an angle problem has occurred. Significant trauma, especially early postoperatively, could also result in displacement of an intraocular lens. The lens position should be verified by wide dilation of the pupil as soon as the anterior chamber is safely reformed. A sudden decompression of trauma may cause peripheral retinal tears, and the patient should be cautioned to report any suspicious symptoms. A retinal consultant should be asked to examine the peripheral part of the retina.

An against-the-rule astigmatism of this magnitude, not predating the surgical intervention, is a surgical emergency. If such a refractive error is allowed to persist, it will nullify in part an otherwise excellent optical result from an intraocular lens, as in this case where the spherical equivalent is -0.50 D. If corrected immediately upon discovery, a simple resuturing after removal of any loosened sutures identified will solve the problem usually without the necessity for a Troutman block or wedge excision of tissue and reconstruction of the wound. I have not discussed the use of Troutman relaxing or other related incisional astigmatism procedures in such cases. They are not indicated because they treat only the symptom and not the basic problem, wound separation.

To influence the degree of postoperative astigmatism during surgery one must first know the keratometry before surgery. A preoperatively flatter vertical corneal meridian will result in an even flatter vertical meridian postoperatively. A preoperatively steeper corneal meridian will tend to be less steep postoperatively. In the latter case, earlier suture removal often will allow even further wound decay toward sphericity. In the case of a flatter vertical corneal meridian, sutures must be left in place longer, any overcorrection must be greater, and when the against-the-rule astigmatism is greater than -2 D, a Troutman wedge or block resection should be done in combination with the corneal incision. I routinely use a clear corneal incision placed vertically through the cornea and closed with full-thickness suture loops. For correction of astigmatism this type of incision is more stable, predictable, and manipulable than is a corneoscleral incision closed with superficially placed sutures. Although the more posteriorly placed incisions initially demonstrate less overcorrection, their inherent instability causes slippage of 2- or 3-D against-the-rule as sutures lose their tensile strength. In shorter incisions, slippage is less, for example, with a 6.5-mm phacoemulsification incision. The longer incision used for manual extracapsular surgery is more prone to delayed wound slippage. If a surgeon who uses a maximum 6.5-mm incision experiences heavy with-the-rule astigmatism from time to time, it is caused by a too-tight suture, detected by photokeratoscopy, and will decay when the suture is cut. Against-the-rule astigmatism, as in our case, is probably due to defective vertical closure, and resuturing under surgical keratometer control is indicated.

A vertical corneal incision closed with Troutman opposing continuous sutures and two interrupted stay sutures should induce approximately 3 D of astigmatism immediately postoperatively. This is released upon removal of the sutures at the end of 12 weeks. If the astigmatism is less than 2 D with the rule after removal of all continuous sutures, one or both of the interrupted stay sutures is left in place indefinitely. If the astigmatism is in excess of 2 D, one or often both sutures are removed. The effective use of a corneal incision requires very deep placement of the closing suture loops, preferably through and through the corneal thickness. This ensures an anatomic reconstruction of the corneal thickness and eliminates unpredictable posterior wound gape as a cause of astigmatism. Such eyes remain stable with astigmatic bands of less than 1 D with the rule after removal of the continuous sutures at 12 weeks. Management of a wound problem in a corneal incision is easier since the internal wound is well anterior to the iris root and the angle is clearly visualized during any repair. In more peripheral incisions where the angle cannot be visualized as well, the iris can be inadvertently included either at the time of the primary suturing or repair. Either type of incision is best made in a single vertical plane so that it can be closed with very short, very deep suture bites inserted with a specially designed needle, the TG6W-C compound-curve needle manufactured by

Ethicon. This needle has a straight, approximately 1-mm pointed end angled into a compound curve of decreasing radius of curvature that becomes almost straight as it approaches the butt of the needle. The needle is driven vertically through the proximal tissue edge, turns quickly to avoid catching iris material beneath the wound, and then is pushed vertically up through the distal tissue edge to create the shortest possible path for a through-and-through loop. In primary or secondary repairs of the cornea the surgeon must keep in mind that the cornea heals from front to back and not from end to end. It is the depth of the closure that determines the strength and integrity of the wound and not the external appearance of closure. Very closely spaced but superficial suture loops do not close a wound. When shallow loops with long bites are used, when tightly tied the internal wound is sprung open, and a posteriorly gaping weakened wound increases the probability of a wound-induced or suture-induced against-the-rule astigmatism such as occurred in the case presented.

Approach 2 ⎯⎯⎯⎯⎯⎯⎯⎯⎯⎯⎯⎯

Jonathan B. Rubenstein, M.D.

This case describes a patient with a resultant high degree of against-the-rule astigmatism after cataract surgery. This is a very frustrating problem that can complicate an otherwise successful surgical procedure. The etiology of this against-the-rule astigmatism is probably secondary to wound slippage or wound gape. There are a multitude of factors that can contribute to wound gape including an anteriorly placed wound, the use of absorbable sutures, postoperative trauma, and the prolonged use of topical steroids.

The refraction in this patient 3 months postoperatively is $-3.00 + 5.00 \times 180$ degrees. It is important to also think of this refraction in its minus cylinder form of $+2.00 - 5.00 \times 90$ degrees. The resulting spherical equivalent is -0.50 D. With this case as an example, this chapter will describe a plan for minimizing postoperative astigmatism through attention to the preoperative and intraoperative situation. Finally, techniques for the surgical correction of astigmatism will be described.

Preoperative Considerations

It is extremely important to pay close attention to the pre-existing astigmatism. Know and understand both the degree and axis of the cylinder. Carefully measure and record preoperative keratometry readings, and determine the exact axis of greatest astigmatism. Perform a careful manifest refraction with special attention to the measurement of astigmatism. If an unusual degree or pattern of astigmatism exists, preoperative photokeratoscopy may also be helpful.

With the knowledge of the preoperative cylinder, plan an approach to cataract surgery that will minimize postoperative astigmatism. Decide on the location of the surgical wound on the basis of the preoperative cylinder. The option is to operate in the axis of greatest plus cylinder vs. operating 90 degrees away. Various investigators have shown that astigmatism may be induced by either wound tightening or wound recession. For example, a cataract patient with a preoperative high degree of astigmatism at 90 degrees could be corrected with a loosely stitched or recessed cataract wound at 90 degrees or a tightly stitched or resected cataract wound via a temporal approach at 180 degrees.

The amount of induced astigmatism is also influenced by the anterior or posterior location of the incision. Most authors have stated that an anteriorly placed incision affects the amount of induced astigmatism to a greater extent than does a posteriorly placed incision. For example, in a patient with a large preoperative degree of with-the-rule astigmatism, a loosely sutured anterior incision at 90 degrees will produce a greater reduction in astigmatism than will a loosely sutured posterior incision at 90 degrees. Alternatively, a posteriorly placed incision probably lessens the chance for high postoperative astigmatism compared with an anteriorly placed incision.

The length of cataract incisions is another variable. Most studies report that shorter incisions induce less astigmatism than do longer incisions. Therefore, one potential benefit from phacoemulsification and small-incision surgery is less surgically induced astigmatism.

The type of suture material and the pattern of suture placement are also important factors in determining postoperative astigmatism. Absorbable sutures such as polyglactin 910 (Vicryl), gut, and chromic are degraded and absorbed 6 to 8 weeks after surgery. Although the initial effect of closure with these sutures is with-the-rule astigmatism secondary to suture tension and tissue edema, the astigmatism eventually shifts to against the rule once the absorbable sutures degrade. Therefore, in order to decrease the chances for postoperative astigmatism in a patient with preoperative with-the-rule astigmatism, the surgeon could close a superiorly placed wound with absorbable sutures.

Closure with nonabsorbable sutures such as nylon usually induces with-the-rule astigmatism. The astigmatism is lessened by suture cutting or by the natural decay of nylon, which occurs after 1 to 2 years. Many studies have shown that selective suture cutting with a nonabsorbable suture can produce very acceptable low degrees of postoperative astigmatism.

Closure may consist of single interrupted sutures or a continuous running suture. The long-term results from either of these techniques are essentially the same. The ultimate effect of either one of these methods probably depends more upon the individual surgeon's technique. The only advantage of individual sutures is the greater degree of postoperative control of astigmatism via individual suture cutting.

My preferred technique, at this time, is to operate on the axis of highest preoperative cylinder. I make a posteriorly placed, scleral pocket incision at the minimum length possible and close the wound with interrupted 10-0 nylon. I selectively cut sutures after 4 weeks when the refractive or keratometric cylinder is greater than 3 D.

Intraoperative Considerations

During surgery, careful attention should be directed toward minimizing postoperative astigmatism. During wound closure, the surgeon must think about tying the sutures at the proper tension. It is important to tie the sutures when the intraocular pressure is in the normal range. Closure with too soft of an eye can produce high astigmatism.

Intraoperative keratometry can be a helpful tool for reducing high postoperative astigmatism. Corneal curvature can be assessed qualitatively with instruments such as a safety pin, a flieringa ring, or a Karickhoff or Troutman keratometer. Quantitative devices like the Terry keratometer can be used as well. Although some studies have shown no significant difference between the astigmatism in eyes closed with or without a surgical keratometer, many authors agree that the keratometer helps to avoid producing very large degrees of postoperative astigmatism. The keratometer also helps the surgeon pay attention to astigmatism and helps develop an awareness of the effects of the individual's suturing technique.

Correction of Astigmatism

Spectacles remain the primary treatment for postoperative astigmatism. The vast majority of cases can be satisfactorily corrected with glasses. When glasses fail, contact lenses should be tried next. Soft toric lenses can correct up to 2.50 D of cylinder. Spherical gas-permeable lenses can correct up to 3.00 D and have the advantage of masking mild degrees of irregular astigmatism. Finally, with a great deal of care and expertise from the fitter, backcurve toric, gas-permeable lenses and speciality lenses such as the Soper lens can correct very high degrees of astigmatism.

When spectacles or contact lenses fail, surgical correction of astigmatism is necessary (Table 4–1). Selective suture cutting is the easiest of these techniques. Suture cutting usually begins between 4 and 8 weeks postoperatively and is performed at the slit lamp with keratometric control. Care must be made to leave a mild degree of residual cylinder with the rule to control for the eventual wound relaxation that occurs months to years later.

Residual high astigmatism that exists after suture manipulation must be handled surgically. The cornea can either be steepened along its flat axis as in a wound revision or wedge resection, or it can be flattened along its steep axis as in relaxing and arcuate incisions, transverse incisions, or trapezoidal keratotomy.

Wound revision is a technique that involves reopening of a slipped or misaligned surgical wound followed by proper wound realignment and resuturing. It is helpful to perform these procedures under the control of a surgical keratometer in order to leave the wound slightly overcorrected at the time of repair.

Another technique that steepens the flat axis is wedge resection. This technique involves the removal of a wedge of corneal tissue down to Descemet's membrane with subsequent tight resuturing of the cornea or limbus in order to affect overall corneal steepening in that meridian. Care is taken not to enter the anterior

TABLE 4–1.

Astigmatic Surgery

Procedure	Range of Effect (D)	Effect on Spherical Equivalence	Comments*
Wedge resection	Up to 27 D Average, ≏ 8D	Variable, tends to induce myopia Steepens the cornea	Long visual rehabilitation Leave sutures 2–6 mo May enter anterior chamber Better for hyperopic astigmatism
Relaxing incisions (+/−) compression sutures	Up to 15 D Usual range, 4.5–8.5	Usually no change	Easier for post-PK Post-PK, at slit lamp Postcataract, in OR with diamond knife
T-cuts	Range, 1–5 D	Usually no change	Easy to quantitate Technically easy ? More predictable
Trapezoidal keratotomy	Range, 1–11 D	Induce hyperopia Overall corneal flattening	Can be done in stepwise fashion to titrate the effect ? More predictable Many clear corneal incisions needed

*OR = operating room; PK = penetrating keratoplasty.

chamber. The length of the excision is usually 90 degrees, with approximately 0.1 mm of corneal tissue excised for every 2 D of correction desired. Usually 7 to 10 sutures are needed to close the wound, and the sutures are tightened to produce an overcorrection of 33% to 50% as measured by a quantitative surgical keratometer. The sutures are selectively removed after a minimum of 2 months until the desired effect is achieved. This procedure steepens the flatter meridian twice as much as it flattens the steep meridian. The overall effect on the spherical equivalent is to induce myopia.

Wedge resections are better suited to postkeratoplasty astigmatism than postcataract astigmatism and have the disadvantage of poor predictability.

Relaxing incisions or arcuate incisions flatten the steep meridian of the cornea. This technique was originally used only for postkeratoplasty astigmatism by making the incisions in the graft-host interface. Arcuate incisions can also be made in clear corneas for postcataract astigmatism. Paired incisions are made 60 to 90 degrees in length, 180 degrees apart along the steep corneal axis. Compression sutures may be added on both sides of the flat axis to increase the effect. Both the arcuate incisions and compression sutures are titrated to produce an overcorrection of approximately 33% when using a surgical keratometer. The steep axis flattens to the same degree that the flat axis steepens, therefore producing no net change in the spherical equivalent.

Transverse incisions (T-cuts) also flatten the steep meridian. These incisions are usually 3 mm long and are made in pairs bordering a 5-mm or a 7-mm optical zone. The incisions are made perpendicular to the steep axis of the cornea. A diamond knife is used to make incisions that penetrate to 80% of the measured corneal thickness. Paired incisions are first made at a 5-mm optical zone. By using intraoperative keratometric guidance, paired incisions may be added at a 7-mm optical zone to increase the flattening affect. These incisions may correct from 1 to 4.5 D of astigmatism depending upon the age of the patient. As in relaxing incisions, the amount of flattening of the steep meridian equals the amount of steepening of the flat meridian, with minimal resulting change in the spherical equivalent.

A procedure with a greater degree of power for flattening the steep meridian is trapezoidal keratotomy. This procedure involves 1 to 2 pairs of transverse incisions made at a 5-mm and a 7-mm or 9-mm optical zone as described earlier and combined with two pairs of semiradial incisions made adjacent to the T-cuts and parallel to the steep axis. The semiradial incisions may extend peripherally from a 3-, 4-, or 5-mm optical zone depending upon the amount of correction desired. As in the T-cuts, incisions are made with a diamond knife to achieve a depth of 80% of the measured corneal thickness. The astigmatic keratotomy may be performed in a stepwise fashion, under intraoperative keratometric control, to titrate the effect to the amount of correction desired in each case. First, paired T-cuts are made at a 5-mm optical zone. If more correction is desired, a second pair of T-cuts are added at a 7-mm or 9-mm optical zone. For more effect, semiradial incisions are added that extend from either a 3-, 4-, or 5-mm optical zone. This procedure can correct 3 to 11 D of astigmatism. Careful attention must be made to center the procedure around the measured axis of astigmatism to avoid changing the axis of astigmatism. This procedure flattens the steep meridian 3 to 4 times as much as it affects the flat meridian, which usually undergoes no change. Therefore the overall affect is to flatten the entire cornea and induce hyperopia. The operation is best suited for eyes with myopic astigmatism where both the myopia and astigmatism can be corrected.

Assuming that spectacle and contact lens corrections have failed, I would approach this case one of two ways. If the surgical wound looked ectatic, I would consider a wound revision with resuturing the wound at the 12-o'clock position. If the wound appeared relatively sound, I would perform transverse incisions in the 180 degree meridian. Using a surgical keratometer, I would begin with paired T-cuts at a 5-mm optical zone. If more correction were needed, I would add a second set of T-cuts at a 7-mm optical zone. The advantage of T-cuts are that they do not change the patient's spherical equivalent. This patient has a spherical equivalent of -0.50 D, which balances well with his other eye, which has a spherical equivalent of -1.00 D. With an ideal result, T-cuts would eliminate most of the 5 D of astigmatism and leave the spherical equivalent near -0.50 D. A trapezoidal keratotomy, alternatively, would leave a spherical equivalent of $+2.00$ D if most of the cylinder were corrected.

These cases of postoperative astigmatism are very difficult to manage. Despite the recent advances made in understanding the surgical correction of astigmatism, these techniques are still often associated with poor predictability and are hindered by a wide variability in effect. Further studies of these techniques and a better knowledge of wound healing will, I hope, increase the accuracy of these procedures in the future.

Bibliography

1. Karickhoff JR: Plus meridian incision for secondary implantation. *Ophthalmic Surg* 1987; 18:658–660.
2. Krachmer JH, Fenzl RE: Surgical correction of high postkeratoplasty astigmatism–relaxing incisions versus wedge resections. *Arch Ophthalmol* 1980; 98:1400–1402.
3. Lindquist TD, Rubenstein JB, Lindstrom RL: Keratotomy for corneal astigmatism. *Semin Ophthalmol* 1986; 1:246–253.
4. Lindquist TD, Rubenstein JB, Rice SW, et al: Trapezoidal astigmatic keratotomy: Quantification in human cadaver eyes. *Arch Ophthalmol* 1986; 104:1534–1539.
5. Lindstrom RL, Destro MA: Effect of incision size and Terry keratometer usage on postoperative astigmatism. *J Am Intraocul Implant Soc* 1985; 11:469–473.
6. Perl T, Binder PS, Earl K: Post-cataract astigmatism with and without the use of the Terry keratometer. *Ophthalmology* 1984; 91:489–493.
7. Swinger CA: Postoperative astigmatism. *Surv Ophthalmol* 1987; 31:219–248.

SECTION II

Cornea and External Disease

Case 5 _____

Epidemic Keratoconjunctivitis— Steer Clear of Steroids?

APPROACH 1

Chandler R. Dawson, M.D.

APPROACH 2

Jonathan B. Rubenstein, M.D.

Case 5 _____

Epidemic Keratoconjunctivitis—
Steer Clear of Steroids?

A 24-year-old nurse had progressive redness, lid swelling, and serous drainage from the right eye for 4 days, at which time the left eye became involved. Now, 1 week later, examination reveals lid swelling and follicular conjunctivitis, and there are subepithelial infiltrates in the right cornea. The visual acuity is 20/60 in the right eye and 20/20 in the left.

The patient is advised against working. She wishes to return to work as soon as possible but does not want to risk a recurrence. What treatment should be offered, and when can she return to work?

Summary

Ophthalmologists fear epidemic keratoconjunctivitis (EKC) because they know that if they catch it they may spend 2 weeks of misery out of the office. When faced with health care workers with EKC there is a temptation to provide whatever treatment will rapidly allow them to return comfortably to work. The question here is whether corticosteroids are that treatment.

Dr. Dawson's approach is conservative and stresses that steroids have never been shown to modify the severity of acute adenovirus eye infections. Most patients should be treated with cold compresses until the body has had an opportunity to eradicate the infection.

After reviewing the typical clinical course, Dr. Rubenstein argues that steroids make patients more comfortable and result in more rapid resolution of the reduced visual acuity associated with the keratitis. They can be used for 1 to 2 weeks and then tapered, reduced in strength, or stopped in order to determine whether the eye will remain quiet without medication.

Both of the discussions stress the importance of ruling out other causes of follicular conjunctivitis that would be worsened by steroids. Of special importance, of course, is herpes simplex virus (HSV) conjunctivitis, which can present in exactly the same way as adenovirus conjunctivitis. However, the subepithelial infiltrates that develop in EKC are characteristic, and in the presence of bilateral disease, HSV is an unlikely diagnosis.

Approach 1 ⎯⎯⎯⎯⎯⎯⎯⎯⎯⎯⎯⎯⎯⎯

Chandler R. Dawson, M.D.

This patient presented with an acute follicular conjunctivitis, first in the right eye and then spreading to the left eye after 4 days. At 1 week after onset there was lid swelling, follicular conjunctivitis, and corneal infiltrates in the right eye, which has a visual acuity of 20/60.

The diagnostic possibilities for this patient's acute follicular conjunctivitis include

- Epidemic keratoconjunctivitis (adenovirus)
- Herpes simplex keratoconjunctivitis
- Adult inclusion conjunctivitis *(Chlamydia trachomatis)*
- *Moraxella* and staphylococcal blepharoconjunctivitis

The laboratory tests that are useful in identifying the problem in order of complexity and cost include

- Giemsa-stained conjunctival smears
- Bacterial cultures of lid margins and conjunctiva
- Fluorescein-labeled monoclonal antibody stain of conjunctival smears (MicroTrak; Syva, Palo Alto, Calif) to detect *C. trachomatis* infection
- Cell cultures or other tests for adenovirus, herpes simplex, or chlamydial agent

Approaches to the Problem: Supportive Therapy Alone

For this problem supportive therapy alone can be used effectively until a definitive diagnosis is obtained that might indicate systemic antibiotic therapy for chlamydial infection. In the cases of viral acute follicular keratoconjunctivitis, therapy consists of cold compresses 3 to 4 times a day to reduce the inflammation and theoretically reduce the replication of virus and extravasation of immune mediators into the tears. Because the occasional staphylococcal or *Moraxella* blepharoconjunctivitis will present in this fashion also, it is a good idea to treat the conjunctiva and lid margins with a topical antibiotic such as erythromycin ointment four times daily.

Patients with this syndrome should be followed closely during the first 2 weeks of the disease. Adenovirus infections will resolve at the end of 2 weeks. During this period of time, patients with follicular conjunctivitis caused by HSV may progress to form dendritiform or other forms of severe keratitis, and they should be treated with the appropriate topical antivirals at that time. A positive herpesvirus culture is also indication for treating with effective antivirals even if a dendritic ulcer has not developed; for patients with only a punctate keratitis the rationale for antiviral treatment is to prevent progression to dendritic or stromal keratitis. If the patient's condition does not clear at 2 weeks after onset, other conditions that might be suspected are keratoconjunctivitis caused by *C. trachomatis*; usually with the sexually transmitted serotypes, staphylococcal lid margin infections are recurrent, and chronic staphylococcal conjunctivitis is often associated with acne rosacea. The chlamydial infections respond to 3 weeks of oral tetracycline or erythromycin in full doses. The staphylococcal blepharitis must be managed with topical medication to the lids, usually erythromycin ointment, lid scrubs, and appropriate shampoos. Patients with acne rosacea receive long-term treatment with oral tetracyclines and are instructed on careful long-term lid hygiene.

For patients suspected of having an adenovirus conjunctivitis who are in the health care field, they should definitely not have any contact with patients for at least 2 weeks after onset. This virus has been recovered from the nasopharynx and eyes for that period of time, and these individuals continue to be infectious and to carry a risk for infecting patients they are caring for.

During the acute phase of the disease topical steroids are definitely contraindicated. Ten percent of these patients with acute follicular conjunctivitis have HSV infection. Treatment with topical steroids enhances the tendency of the virus to involve the cornea, stroma, and uveal tract during the acute phase. There is no controlled trial to show that topical corticosteroids are useful in modifying the severity of acute adenovirus eye infections. Indeed, if one takes the analogy with herpesvirus, steroid treatment may actually enhance the ability of the virus to proliferate in the conjunctival and corneal epithelium and thus produce more long-term damage.

If this patient goes on to develop typical anterior stromal opacities of EKC, the primary indication for steroid treatment to suppress these opacities is the patient's inability to perform visual tasks needed for their life. If the vision is definitely diminished and the patient needs vision in the eye, a low concentration of corticosteroid such as prednisolone acetate $1/_8$% can be started four times a day. If the opacities resolve on this treatment, the steroid dose may be progressively decreased to the point where the opacities do not reappear within a week at the next lower dose. Patients must often be maintained on a very low dose of steroids for several months. The resolution of EKC opacities is extremely variable. Many patients develop no opacities at all or have only a few. Even in those patients with many opacities they will often resolve in 3 to 4 months. Thus patients who are receiving steroid treatment must be tested from time to time by discontinuing topical steroid treatment and following the patient for the recurrence of the opacities.

Again, topical corticosteroids are absolutely contraindicated in any patient who has had an ocular herpes virus infection.

If the MicroTrak or other test for *Chlamydia* is positive, the patient should receive treatment with oral tetracycline (or alternatively, oral erythromycin) in full systemic doses for 3 weeks. Particularly with a positive laboratory test result for *Chlamydia*, treatment of the patient's sexual consort or consorts at the same time should be discussed with the patient. *C trachomatis* infections are particularly dangerous for women because fallopian tubes become infected and the disease may progress to stricture of the fallopian tubes and sterility.

For contact lens wearers it is always a difficult point to decide when the patient should start wearing contact lenses again. In most cases it is a good idea to wait until the epithelial lesions have resolved and there is a good idea of what the density of corneal opacities will be. There is no evidence that wearing soft lenses exacerbates the opacities or enhances the tendency for corneal erosions.

Approach 2

Jonathan B. Rubenstein, M.D.

This case describes a bilateral, asymmetrical case of acute conjunctivitis in a young individual who works in a health care setting. The conjunctivitis leads to a keratitis 11 days later. This scenario is typical for EKC secondary to an adenoviral infection. Using this case as an example, this chapter will provide a brief discussion of the etiology, pathogenesis, clinical features, laboratory diagnosis, and management of EKC. Special emphasis will be placed on the role of corticosteroids in the management of this disease.

EKC is a type of acute keratoconjunctivitis caused by the adenovirus. Multiple types of adenovirus have been shown to be associated with this disease, including types 1 to 11, 13 to 16, 19, and 29. Types 8 and 19 are presently the most common adenovirus types associated with EKC in the United States.

EKC is of great concern to the ophthalmologist because of the ease of transmission of this virus through direct contact in a hospital or physician's office. The affected individual, in this case example, is a nurse who probably works in a setting that puts her at a greater risk for contracting an adenoviral infection. The transmission of virus is usually from contaminated fingers, solutions, or instruments. Many epidemics have been linked to the contaminated hands or instruments of ophthalmologists and the assistants in an ophthalmologist's office. Devices such as tonometers and trial contact lenses are often vectors of transmission. Therefore, adequate hand washing and cleansing and sterilization of ophthalmic instruments between patient examinations is extremely important. Adenovirus may also be spread in the community by close personal or sexual contact. Community epidemics have also been linked to a common exposure to swimming pools. The incubation period for the virus is an average of 8 days, with a range of 2 to 16 days (Fig 5–1).

The initial clinical manifestation of the disease is as an acute follicular conjunctivitis. The disease starts in only one eye, with the second eye becoming involved approximately 4 to 5 days later. The conjunctivitis is predominantly follicular, yet a papillary response often overlies the follicles. There is an associated watery discharge and swollen, tender preauricular lymph nodes, worse on the side of the first eye involved. Pseudomembranes with resultant symblepharon formation may occur in up to one third of cases. Conjunctival involvement lasts from 7 to 14 days, yet corneal involvement lasts longer. Initially, the cornea shows the pres-

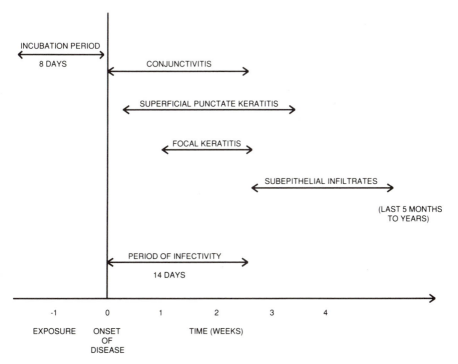

FIG 5–1.
Time course of clinical features and infectivity of EKC.

ence of a fine superficial punctate keratitis that stains with fluorescein dye. Between the 7th and 13th days, the areas of superficial keratitis coalesce to form larger areas of focal keratitis. In at least one half of these cases, subepithelial infiltrates (SEIs) appear just beneath the areas of focal keratitis. The subepithelial opacities usually appear between the 14th and 20th day and may persist for months to many years. The opacities represent sensitized T lymphocytes that are attracted to a viral protein or inactive virion. The SEIs may be quite debilitating by causing a significant degree of photophobia and a significant decrease in visual acuity if centrally located. Some patients may also exhibit a mild anterior uveitis that accompanies their focal keratitis. Live virus may be isolated up to 14 days after the onset of the disease. Therefore, patients with EKC remain infectious for 2 weeks after the onset of symptoms.

The diagnosis of adenoviral infection may be made in one of four ways. A Giemsa stain of a conjunctival scraping will show a predominately mononuclear response. Patients with pseudomembranes will also have a significant number of polymorphonuclear leukocytes. Virus may be isolated via cell culture, yet positive results may take 3 to 4 weeks. Blood tests will reveal a fourfold increase in antibody titers between acute and convalescent sera. The best method of identifying adenovirus is with fluorescent-antibody staining of conjunctival smears. This technique provides a simple, reliable, and rapid method of diagnosis.

The treatment of EKC is somewhat controversial. Everyone agrees that relative isolation of affected patients is advisable. Measures that limit the spread of the disease must be taught to infected individuals. Patients should carefully wash their hands after touching their eyes, should avoid the use of shared towels and linens, and should avoid kissing and direct oral contact with other people. Because they may remain infectious for 14 days, people with EKC should stay home from work for 2 weeks after contracting the disease. The nurse in our case, as a person who comes in direct contact with many people while working, should stay away from work for 2 weeks.

Often symptomatic treatment with topical decongestant eye drops and cold compresses are enough to make some patients comfortable. In general, patients should be given the least amount of medicine that is necessary to maintain an adequate degree of comfort.

Unfortunately, none of the currently available antiviral medications has been found to be clinically effective in managing EKC. Trials with topical human fibroblast interferon are currently being studied.

Corticosteroid therapy represents the core of controversy surrounding the treatment of EKC. Opponents of steroid therapy maintain that these drugs prolong the course of an otherwise self-limited disease. The indications for steroid therapy are twofold. In those cases with a severe conjunctival reaction producing pseudomembranes, topical steroid therapy provides a dramatic reduction in the inflammatory response and therefore leads to regression of the pseudomembranes and a lessened chance of symblepharon formation. Many patients with subepithelial corneal opacities suffer a significant loss of visual acuity. These people often have a disabling degree of photophobia and discomfort as well. This is the other group of patients who are helped by corticosteroids. Topical steroids will rapidly cause the SEIs to disappear. Because the natural course of the disease is chronic, steroid therapy may have to be continued at a low dose for months to years to suppress the presence of SEIs. It must be remembered that corticosteroids do not alter the basic pathogenetic mechanisms of the disease, they only suppress its signs. Care must also be given to only treat with steroids when the presence of other causes of follicular conjunctivitis like HSV and *Chlamydia* have been ruled out because steroids may worsen the course of these diseases.

In our case of the 24-year-old nurse, I would treat with topical steroids once the SEIs appeared if their presence caused a disabling degree of photophobia or decreased visual acuity. I would give 1% prednisolone acetate drops four times a day until symptoms improve to a level that permits the patient the opportunity to function normally. This usually takes 1 to 2 weeks. Then I would taper the dose as rapidly as possible until reaching a low maintenance dose. Often patients can function on doses of 0.125% prednisolone acetate every other day. Stopping treatment with the drops should be tried periodically to determine whether the patient can function without medicine. The end point is to have a patient who can resume a normal life-style, not necessarily a cornea that is free of opacities.

Bibliography

1. Dawson CR, et al: Adenovirus type 8 keratoconjunctivitis in the United States: III. Epidemiologic, clinical, and microbiologic features. *Am J Ophthalmol* 1970; 69:473.
2. Grayson M: Acute and Chronic Follicular Conjunctivitis, in Grayson M (ed): *Diseases of the Cornea*. St Louis, CV Mosby Co, 1979.
3. Laibson PR, et al: Corneal infiltrates in epidemic keratoconjunctivitis: Response to double-blind corticosteroid therapy. *Arch Ophthalmol* 1970; 84:36–40.
4. Leibowitz HM: *Corneal Disorders: Clinical Diagnosis and Management*. Philadelphia,WB Saunders Co, 1984, pp 234–235.
5. Smolin G, Thoft RA: *The Cornea: Scientific Foundations and Clinical Practice*. Boston, Little, Brown & Co, Inc, 1983, pp 196–209.

Case 6 _____

Episcleritis and Scleritis—Which Drugs Are Indicated?

APPROACH 1

Robert S. Dawson, M.D.

APPROACH 2

Robert A. Nozik, M.D.

Case 6 ⎯⎯⎯⎯⎯⎯⎯⎯⎯⎯⎯

Episcleritis and Scleritis—Which Drugs Are Indicated?

A 50-year-old woman has had redness near the temporal limbus of her left eye for 10 days. It is locally tender, but her main complaint is the unsightly appearance. Examination is normal except for a localized area of inflammation that is interpreted as episcleritis. Her medical history is positive for rheumatoid arthritis, and she currently takes indomethacin, 50 mg three times a day.

The patient is distressed by her condition and seeks rapid resolution. What treatment options are available?

Summary _____

Localized areas of epibulbar inflammation are annoying and sometimes painful. Patients are typically young and active and want
rapid resolution. Proper management requires an understanding
of the differential diagnosis and the numerous treatment options.

Dr. Weinberg discusses the differentiation between episcleritis
and scleritis. He then outlines a sequential approach to management that ranges from observation to cytotoxic agents. It is important that the physician and patient understand the implications
of each of the treatment options before embarking on therapy.

The management of episcleritis is emphasized by Dr. Nozik.
He favors a conservative approach since the disease is self-limited
and is usually only a cosmetic problem. He mentions flurbiprofen
(Ocufen), a new nonsteroidal anti-inflammatory agent that might
have some effect in this condition.

Both discussions center around the importance of making the
right diagnosis. As in many conditions, if the patient does not
improve within 2 to 3 weeks, the physician should entertain the
possibility that the wrong diagnosis has been made. At that point,
a further workup might be in order for looking for other causes
of localized epibulbar inflammation.

Approach 1

Robert A. Nozik, M.D.

In discussing the management of this patient's ocular inflammation, the first thing to establish is the diagnosis.

Differential Diagnosis

In this case the only important considerations are phlyctenulosis, scleritis, pingueculitis, and episcleritis.

Phlyctenulosis

This condition, which appears as a focal (nodular) inflammation at or on either side of the corneal scleral junction, is characterized by considerable pain. Also there is necrosis and ulceration of the elevated nodule at the center of the inflammation. Since neither severe pain nor ulceration is present in this patient, we can eliminate phlyctenulosis as the diagnosis in this case.

Scleritis

Scleritis, which may be either nodular or diffuse, is a very painful condition. Often it is associated with inflammation of the deep sclera and underlying uvea that results in secondary anterior uveitis or serous detachment of the ciliary body or choroid, depending on the location of the scleritis. The scleral injection, while often a bright, diffuse redness, will usually also include a bluish or violet color indicating deep scleral inflammation. Often areas of sclera will show bluish thinning as a result of prior necrotizing attacks of scleritis. In the case presented, the lack of severe pain, absence of scleral thinning, and absence of secondary uveal inflammation eliminates scleritis as the primary inflammatory process.

Pingueculitis

Pingueculitis may be considered a variant of nodular episcleritis. The injection is centered about the area of the pinguecula and is primarily a cosmetic problem. There may be mild discomfort, but this is never severe. The lack of the notation of a pinguecula in this case eliminates this diagnosis.

Episcleritis

Episcleritis involves inflammation of the loose vascular tissue situated between the sclera and the conjunctiva. The pattern may be nodular or diffuse. When it is nodular, there is an elevated, focal inflammation, often associated with minimal pain. Diffuse episcleritis is usually limited to one quadrant, relatively flat in appearance, and minimally painful. Episcleritis usually occurs near the limbus, often in the palpebral fissure area.

The case presented, based on the aforementioned descriptions, represents a case of diffuse episcleritis.

Disease Associations in Episcleritis

Next we must decide whether or not to do any diagnostic workup in this case.

Most cases (approximately 70%) of episcleritis fail to reveal any associated disease and are considered to represent an autoimmune disease state. Conditions that have been associated with episcleritis include connective tissue diseases, especially rheumatoid arthritis and gout, and systemic infections such as herpes zoster, herpes simplex, Epstein-Barr virus, tuberculosis, syphilis, coccidioidomycosis, and chronic staphylococcal infections. Other systemic associates include Wegener's granulomatosis, Crohn's disease, Hansen's disease, and certain forms of glomerulonephritis.

I believe that no workup is indicated in the present case since she already carries the diagnosis of rheumatoid arthritis and her episcleritis is most likely associated with this.

Course and Sequelae

Episcleritis is a benign inflammation and does not lead to significant ocular damage. Less than 15% of cases may develop mild thinning and opacification of the adjacent cornea. It is primarily a cause of mild irritation and cosmetic annoyance. Also, except for episcleritis associated with herpes zoster, it does not tend to progress to scleritis.

Most cases last a total of 10 to 20 days before resolving spontaneously. Treatment generally does not shorten the course of the disease but may reduce the symptoms of discomfort and redness.

Management

Immunosuppressives and systemic corticosteroids can be dispensed with quickly. While these potent anti-inflammatory agents would be effective, their very significant and potentially severe side effects eliminate their use in such a benign inflammation as episcleritis.

Topical corticosteroids, strong or weak, will reduce the episcleral inflammation but do carry the risk of significant and well-known complications. These include secondary glaucoma, cataract, and potentiation of infection.

Nonsteroidal anti-inflammatory agents, topical or systemic, are often useful in reducing episcleral inflammation.

Whitening agents (vasoconstrictors) do little to reduce the actual episcleral inflammation but do minimize the redness for cosmetic improvement.

Summary

This patient's episcleritis is probably related to her rheumatoid arthritis. If she has minimal symptoms and rapid resolution, I would do no further workup.

Since her main concern is the cosmetic appearance, I would treat her with whitening agents to reduce redness. She is already taking systemic indomethacin, which should help in reducing the inflammation. Topical indomethacin or the new agent Ocufen could be tried in this case, or even a mild topical steroid. Since this is a benign, self-limited disease, I would resist the use of strong topical or any systemic steroids.

Bibliography

1. Allansmith MR: *The Eye and Immunology*. St Louis, CV Mosby Co, 1982, pp 142–144.
2. Ostler HB, Dawson CR, Okumoto M: *Color Atlas of Infections and Inflammatory Diseases of the External Eye*. Baltimore, Urban & Schwarzenberg, 1987, p 104.
3. Smolin G, and O'Connor GR: *Ocular Immunology*, ed 2. Boston, Little, Brown & Co, Inc, 1986, pp 229–231.
4. Smolin G, Thoft RA (eds): *The Cornea*. Boston, Little, Brown & Co, Inc, 1983, p 253.
5. Watson PG, Hayreh SS: Scleritis and episcleritis. *Br J Ophthalmol* 1976; 60:167–191.

Approach 2 _____

Robert S. Weinberg, M.D.

In a patient with rheumatoid arthritis, ocular involvement is not uncommon. Most often the ocular involvement takes the form of keratitis sicca, with complaints of redness of the eyes and foreign body sensation. When the redness is localized, either episcleritis or scleritis may be present. Either or both can occur in patients with rheumatoid arthritis. Although there are exceptions to the typical presentation, the symptoms and signs of episcleritis and scleritis differ. So too does the management. It is important therefore to be certain of the diagnosis prior to recommending treatment.

To aid in understanding the difference between episcleritis and scleritis, a knowledge of the anatomy is necessary. The episclera is a vascularized layer of connective tissue contiguous but superficial to the sclera. At the limbus, the episclera is adherent to overlying Tenon's capsule, which lies under the conjunctiva. Tenon's capsule is thicker anteriorly than posteriorly and consists of collagen fibrils that are radially oriented. Episcleral collagen fibrils are circumferentially oriented. There are few nerve fibers in the episclera, hence the usual absence of pain as a symptom of episcleritis.

Scleral collagen fibrils vary in size, with both superficial and deep layers. At the limbus the fibers are circumferential, but posteriorly there is a netlike pattern, except near the macula where there is a circular pattern. There are many nerve fibers in the sclera, which accounts for the pain of scleral inflammation. Scleral stroma normally contains no blood vessels, with nutrition supplied by episcleral and choroidal vessels. The anterior ciliary arteries supply the episclera and Tenon's capsule anteriorly; the posterior ciliary arteries supply blood to the episclera and Tenon's capsule posterior to the rectus in sections.[1]

78

Episcleritis

Typically the patient with episcleritis is a woman from 20 to 50 years of age. There may be minimal watery discharge from the eye, but usually there is no change in vision. Pain may be present, but usually it is not. Injection may be diffuse or localized. If localized, the area of involvement may be extensive enough to give a nodular appearance, hence the term *nodular episcleritis*. Nodular episcleritis is much less common than is diffuse episcleritis. On examination the area of involvement may be bright red or deep pink in color. The area of inflammation may or may not be tender to the touch. With the aid of a cotton-tipped applicator, the area of episcleritis can be movable over deeper tissues.

If there is true episcleritis confirmed by clinical examination, then there are four alternatives to management. The first alternative would be simple observation, with the realization that episcleritis is not a destructive or vision-threatening process. If the problem has not resolved, however, within approximately 7 to 10 days, some form of therapeutic intervention is usually requested by the patient. The second approach would be simply to use topical decongestant agents. This does not eliminate the problem but may give some cosmetic improvement. Such agents as naphazoline hydrochloride, 0.1%, may be used four times a day for several days to decrease vascular congestion. The third approach would be to use topical corticosteroids frequently. Either fluorometholone, prednisolone acetate, or dexamethasone phosphate can be effective in relieving the local inflammation from episcleritis. In general, the beginning dose should range from four times a day to every 2 hours depending on the extent and severity of the lesion. Treatment with topical corticosteroids should be continued for 7 to 10 days or at least for several days after resolution of objective signs of inflammation. The fourth approach would be to use systemic agents. In this particular patient in the example, systemic antiprostaglandin therapy has already been instituted. The use of these drugs would generally be the first line of approach in the use of systemic medications. If a patient is already taking systemic antiprostaglandin agents, increasing the dosage can be helpful. In general, there is little increased efficacy to be gained by switching from one agent to another agent in this category. Systemic corticosteroids then are the last method of approach. Systemic corticosteroids in the form of prednisone in a dose of 40 to 60 mg a day can accomplish resolution of the local inflammation of episcleritis. Most often, however, the condition is not severe enough to warrant the use of systemic corticosteroid medications.

Episcleritis tends to be self-limited. There is generally no pain and no change in visual acuity. For that reason a conservative approach is advisable. In the patient who is significantly affected by the cosmetic appearance, the least amount of therapy that can accomplish a resolution of the problem is advisable.

Scleritis

Scleritis may be diffuse or nodular and extensive or localized. Pain is a frequent symptom, and often the pain is severe. Localized tenderness detectable on examination with gentle pressure with a cotton-tipped applicator may be a helpful clinical sign. Vascular congestion imparts a dark red or purple color. However, the most difficult differential is between nodular episcleritis and nodular scleritis. In the latter, pain and localized tenderness are common findings.

If the localized limbal lesion is a true scleritis, there are several alternatives to management. In general, topical agents are not effective in producing resolution of a localized scleritis. Topical agents may be of some value in increasing comfort, but almost invariably systemic agents are required. Periocular injections of corticosteroids are controversial. There is some concern that periocular corticosteroid administration may cause localized scleral thinning and therefore are contraindicated in a process in which the end result may be a localized scleral destruction. In a patient with rheumatoid arthritis, a posterior injection may be dangerous because of localized scleral staphylomas located posteriorly that may not be obvious when examining the eye anteriorly.

The therapeutic approach to localized scleritis, or diffuse scleritis for that matter, should begin with the least dangerous agents and progress to more toxic drugs if the weaker drugs do not accomplish resolution of the process. In general in the typical patient with scleritis, pain relief occurring within 48 to 96 hours of institution of the appropriate systemic agent will be the first sign of effectiveness of therapy.

I will generally begin with systemic indomethacin. The dose of systemic indomethacin ranges from 25 mg two or three times a day to 75 mg twice a day. Indomethacin appears to be more effective in decreasing scleral inflammation than other, newer, less gastrointestinal-irritating antiprostaglandin agents. In addition, the general ophthalmic experience with the newer agents is much less extensive than that with indomethacin, which has been available for some time. In a patient who is already taking indomethacin as the patient in this example, increasing the systemic indomethacin to a higher tolerated dose would be the first approach recommended. If after 4 to 7 days there has not been resolution, then one can consider going to the next line of drugs, which would be systemic corticosteroids. Before beginning systemic indomethacin treatment, the patient must be warned of the gastrointestinal side effects of heartburn and nausea that may occasionally occur. In patients with a history of peptic ulcer disease antacids may be instituted early.

When systemic antiprostaglandin agents are not effective, systemic corticosteroids generally are. Prednisone in a dose of 40 to 60 mg a day is usually effective in causing decreased scleral inflammation and in those patients with pain, resolution of the pain. Occasionally in a patient with diffuse scleritis doses of 80 to 120 mg of prednisone a day may be necessary. Such high doses have an increased likelihood of side effects such as hyperglycemia and fluid retention, but for a short period of time those side effects may be managed. I prefer to use prednisone in a dose of 40 to 60 mg per day in one dose for 7 days and then begin tapering the dose after there has been a response. Systemic corticosteroids should be continued for at least 4 or more days after resolution of the acute ocular inflammation. Tapering of the systemic corticosteroid can be done over several weeks if the drug can be discontinued in the patient.

While systemic corticosteroids are the second line of therapeutic approach in managing localized or diffuse scleritis in the majority of patients, in some patients avoidance of corticosteroid usage should be considered. In the patient who has been unresponsive to high doses of systemic corticosteroids or in the insulin-dependent diabetic, the use of immunosuppressive agents should be considered if antiprostaglandin agents are not effective. Many ophthalmologists are not familiar with the usage of these drugs, and working closely with a rheumatologist or oncologist in the management of patients receiving systemic immunosuppressive agents is frequently advisable. In managing localized or diffuse scleritis, cyclophosphamide (Cytoxan) or azathioprine (Imuran) are most commonly employed. Chlorambucil has been utilized in the management of some types of scleritis, but in general because the use of chlorambucil requires a slow increase in dosage to achieve a therapeutic effect, the time required for decreased inflammation secondary to chlorambucil treatment is usually longer than that required for Cytoxan or Imuran. Imuran has been associated in some instances with late-onset lymphoma but still is effective in the management of the many connective tissue diseases and in scleritis. The dose of Imuran is 50 to 100 mg per day. Periodic white blood counts and platelet counts should be obtained to avoid hematologic complications of this drug. Cytoxan in a dose of 50 to 200 mg per day is extremely effective in obtaining resolution of scleral inflammation. In general the patient will have decreased subjective evidence of inflammation, with decreased pain within several days. Objective evidence of resolution with decreased injection and inflammation may lag behind by several days. Any patient placed on a regimen of Cytoxan should be warned of the hematologic side effects, which include leukopenia and thrombocytopenia. Cystitis in a hemorrhagic form can be quite troublesome, and adequate fluid intake should be recommended. Frequent white blood counts and platelet counts should be monitored to prevent leukopenia and thrombocytopenia. Once there has been a significant fall in a white cell count or a platelet count, the dose of Cytoxan should be cut back or treatment with the drug should be discontinued altogether.

Once Cytoxan treatment has been started, therapy should be continued until the objective signs of inflammation have decreased. The patient may be left with an area of scleromalacia, even though this was not evident in the initial presentation. The aim of therapy is decreased discomfort, preservation of vision, and preservation of the integrity of the globe.

New forms of therapy and older forms of therapy have been investigated in the treatment of localized scleritis. In patients who have rheumatoid arthritis, systemic gold therapy has not proved to be effective in decreasing scleral inflammation, although it certainly may be effective in controlling signs and symptoms of the articular components of the disease. Plasmapheresis has been used occasionally for the systemic complications of rheumatoid arthritis. Intravenous pulse therapy with high-dose methylprednisolone has been advised by some authors for the management of scleritis.[2] High-dose intravenous pulse therapy for scleritis generally requires hospitalization. Systemic side effects may occur, but initial reports suggest that there can be excellent resolution of ocular inflammation with large doses of intravenous methylprednisolone acetate. In general, patients with scleritis even more severe than in the patient in this example do not require hospitalization either for evaluation or therapy.

In this patient, then, with known rheumatoid arthritis and localized disease with excellent vision and minimal pain, conservative management is advisable. It is important to be able to differentiate localized nodular episcleritis from true scleritis, for the management of the two conditions is not the same. Patient education and reassurance is extremely helpful in long-term management of these patients, particularly the patient with rheumatoid arthritis who is likely to have significant and possibly severe ocular involvement the longer the disease is present. Approaching these patients in an organized fashion, confirming the diagnosis, and treating with the least toxic agents initially is recommended.

References

1. Watson PG, Hagleman BL: *The Sclera and Systemic Disorders.* London, WB Saunders Co, Ltd, 1976, pp 15–23.
2. McCluskey P, Wakefield D: Intravenous pulse methylprednisolone in scleritis. *Arch Ophthalmol* 1987; 105:793–797.

Dendritic Keratitis— Will Wiping It Off Wipe It Out?

APPROACH 1

Randy J. Epstein, M.D.

APPROACH 2

Kirk R. Wilhelmus, M.D.

Case 7 ———————————

Dendritic Keratitis—Will Wiping It Off Wipe It Out?

A 37-year-old business executive complains of having had a red left eye for the past 3 days. Examination finds 20/40 vision, moderate injection of the conjunctiva, and a small, paracentral dendritic corneal ulcer.

What is the best approach to diagnosis and treatment?

Summary _____

The problem presented by this case is the controversy over whether debridement alone is as effective as the addition or substitution of antiviral medications, particularly in what appears to be the first instance of dendritic keratitis. The expense and inconvenience of medications argue in favor of debridement alone, but what do the experts do?

Debridement is useful in obtaining a specimen for culture, and Dr. Epstein favors it for this reason. However, he points out that there is evidence that debridement followed by the use of an antiviral agent promotes more rapid healing than the antiviral medication used without debridement.

Dr. Wilhelmus points out that the available studies have yielded conflicting results, with some reports showing more rapid epithelialization by 1 to 2 days when debridement is added to topical therapy. This may not seem to be a clinically significant advantage, but he reminds us that epithelial healing re-establishes the protective surface barrier and reduces symptoms. If this minimizes lost time from work or school, then even a short increase in healing rate would be beneficial.

Both experts stress the importance of laboratory diagnosis in cases of dendritic keratitis. Even when the clinical appearance is classic, only three quarters of these lesions are culture-positive. These diagnostic tools should be used in order to guard against allowing patients to be incorrectly labeled as having a "history of herpes keratitis."

Approach 1 _____

Randy J. Epstein, M.D.

The case under discussion involves a 37-year-old with a 3-day history of a red eye and a dendritic corneal ulcer. While the most likely diagnosis in this case, if the lesion is indeed a "true dendrite," is acute epithelial herpes simplex keratitis, this case presents an opportunity to discuss the differential diagnosis of dendriform corneal lesions.

Differential Diagnosis

Tooma and associates presented a series of 29 cases of dendriform corneal lesions at the 1984 meeting of the American Academy of Ophthalmology. These included 17 cases of herpes simplex keratitis, 7 cases of herpes zoster and/or epithelial mucus plaques, 2 related to contact lens wear, 2 healing epithelial defects, and 1 from a recurrent corneal erosion. One other entity associated with corneal dendriform lesions, not noted in this study, is systemic tyrosinemia.

Corneal lesions associated with herpes zoster, recently reviewed,[1] include "pseudodendrites." These lesions are rarely associated with frank corneal ulceration. They consist of elevated areas of swollen epithelial cells that have club-shaped tips and are much narrower than are the lesions associated with herpes simplex. Frequently, these lesions are associated with overlying mucus plaques. Mucus plaques can also occur in the absence of dendriform lesions. Patients with corneal involvement from herpes zoster generally have profoundly and diffusely decreased corneal sensation.

Dendriform lesions associated with contact lens wear should be suspected in any patient with the appropriate history.[2] These lesions are rarely ulcerated and thus cause pooling rather than staining with fluorescein dye. It has been suggested that they are related to toxicity or hypersensitivity to contact lens solutions and/or preservatives.[3] They generally resolve following temporary discontinuation of contact lens wear and a change in disinfection methods.

Healing epithelial defects, if seen a number of days after the original injury, can frequently have a dendriform appearance. This is due to the "seams" that are formed by palisading epithelial cells, which cause pooling of fluorescein around the elevated area. These lesions will usually resolve within a couple of days without treatment. Healing epithelial defects related to recurrent corneal erosions have an elevated, heaped-up appearance, frequently associated with negative fluorescein staining or pooling. Areas of recurrent erosion can be identified, even when no staining is seen, by gentle indentation and applying a cotton-tipped applicator to the area of suspicious epithelium after the instillation of a topical anesthetic. If an area of recurrent erosion is present, the epithelium will slide easily over the surface of the cornea because it is poorly adherent to the underlying Bowman's layer due to faulty or excessive production of basement membrane.

Finally, tyrosinemia is also associated with dendriform lesions in the cornea. These lesions are seen with systemic tyrosinemia, type 2. They are slightly elevated and stain irregularly with fluorescein. They are usually bilateral and generally seen in children. The diagnosis can be established by the presence of elevated levels of tyrosine and its metabolites in the serum and urine.[2]

Herpes Simplex Dendritic Keratitis: Diagnosis

If the lesion is truly a dendrite caused by herpes simplex virus, it should exhibit intense staining with rose bengal dye (which stains dead or devitalized cells) and positive staining with fluorescein (which stains basement membranes), especially in the central ulcerated area. The lesion generally causes a depression in the surface of the cornea. It is characterized by extensive arborization, with the tips of the lesion terminating in "bulbs." Decreased corneal sensation is frequently localized to the area of the dendrite, while the surrounding corneal sensation can remain normal. It is easily assessed subjectively by touching the area of the dendrite with the finely pulled tip of a sterile cotton applicator. Patients with dendritic herpes simplex dendritic keratitis frequently have a recent history of "cold sores" around the eyes or mouth. Primary herpes simplex infections present either as an upper respiratory tract infection, cold sores around the eyes or mouth, acute follicular conjunctivitis, or dendritic keratitis.[4] Any patient with a unilateral, acute follicular conjunctivitis should be suspected of having herpes simplex virus until proved otherwise. Up to 23% of patients with acute conjunctivitis in a large British series were found to harbor herpes simplex virus.[4] Furthermore, herpes simplex blepharoconjunctivitis can present bilaterally. Therefore, one is not safe treating a patient with acute follicular conjunctivitis with steroids until the patient has been followed for a sufficient length of time to allow exclusion of this diagnosis. The consequences of treating acute epithelial herpetic disease with topical corticosteroids can be devastating.

In addition to its morphological features and associated clinical findings, dendritic herpes simplex keratitis can be diagnosed with certainty by using a number of laboratory methods. One of the more widely available tests is the viral culture. Most hospital laboratories perform this test routinely and can handle eye specimens. I like to perform general debridement of the lesions with a Virocult swab (Medical Wire & Equipment Co, Ltd, Potley, Corsham, Wilts, England). Following instillation of a topical anesthetic, the swab is used to gently remove the entire dendrite. Usually the lesion is well circumscribed and easily removed, with minimal disturbance to the surrounding, uninvolved cells. This specimen is then sent to the laboratory for viral culture after placing it on ice. This not only allows one to collect a specimen for culture and diagnosis, but it also achieves a therapeutic objective, debridement. In a recent study, debridement was compared with debridement plus trifluorothymidine and trifluorothymidine alone.[5] Both of the latter two groups were found to have significantly faster healing rates, with fewer treatment failures than in patients treated with debridement alone. There was not, however, any difference between the groups treated with debridement plus antiviral and the group treated with antiviral alone. Nonetheless, prior to the advent of topical antivirals, debridement was the only available treatment for dendritic corneal ulcers. The elimination of actively replicating virus is easily accomplished. This may result in either a more rapid cure or a diminished frequency of recurrences, although this has not been proved conclusively. It can be argued that if done too vigorously this technique may damage Bowman's layer and make the patient more susceptible to recurrent corneal erosions. A technique has recently been described in which impression cytology paper strips are used to perform the debridement.[6] This technique is felt by the authors to effect a more complete removal of infected epithelial cells while disturbing the surrounding normal cells to a lesser extent. I also like to perform debridement because one is able to send a specimen to the laboratory for a definitive diagnosis. Viral cultures are positive in up to 78% of these cases.[7] Many patients are followed for years with only a clinical diagnosis of herpes simplex keratitis. Some patients who have been followed on this basis have recently been found to have *Acanthamoeba* keratitis, and were subjected to inappropriate therapy, sometimes for months, because of misdiagnosis.[8] Therefore, it behooves the clinician to make this diagnosis with certainty when the opportunity presents itself.

Other techniques for making the diagnosis of herpes simplex keratitis include the use of immunofluorescent antibody staining of corneal scrapings.[7] This technique has the advantage of being extremely rapid, and it is currently being investigated as a cost-effective diagnostic tool for general utilization. At the present time, however, it is restricted to centers with fluorescence microscopy facilities. Viral particles can also be seen by transmission electron microscopy.

A patient who presents with acute dendritic keratitis has a 25% chance of stromal disease developing, with 75% of these cases occurring in the first year.[9] Once a patient has suffered a second episode of dendritic keratitis, there is a 48% chance of recurrent disease developing. The pathogenesis, diagnosis, and treatment of stromal herpetic disease is beyond the scope of this discussion.

Herpes Simplex Dendritic Keratitis: Treatment

The ideal treatment of a dendrite kills the virus and/or removes infected cells and lessens the likelihood of stromal disease developing. In animals inoculated with live herpes virus, if antiviral therapy was initiated within the first week, there was a lower incidence of stromal disease than animals that were not treated within the first week.[10] It is currently accepted that trifluorothymidine is the drug of choice in the treatment of acute dendritic keratitis in the United States.[11] This drug is generally administered every 2 hours while the patient is awake, or 7 to 9 times per day. The dosage is subsequently tapered if the patient shows the appropriate clinical response. In Great Britain where topical acyclovir has been approved for ophthalmic use, it has been shown to have comparable but not superior efficacy when compared with trifluorothymidine.[9] Acyclovir has the significant advantage of being taken up only by cells infected with replicating virus and not by uninfected cells. Nonetheless, trifluorothymidine is a relatively nontoxic drug, especially when compared with some of the older antivirals such as idoxuridine (IDU), and viral resistance is rare.

It is also important to distinguish between recurrent dendritic ulceration and persistent epithelial defects/recurrent erosions that result from incomplete healing of the epithelium, also known as metaherpetic keratitis. Metaherpetic keratitis is usually associated with significantly decreased corneal sensation. Treatment is largely supportive, including the use of lubricants and therapeutic bandage contact lenses.

In summary, for this patient, I would recommend Virocult debridement followed by immediate topical trifluorothymidine every 2 hours while awake until the lesion is healed. I would send the specimen to the laboratory for viral culture. If the culture was positive, I would counsel the patient that he had up to a 25% chance of recurrence, most likely within the first year, and I would warn him to call the office quickly should he develop signs of ocular irritation after the initial episode had subsided.

References

1. Liesegang TJ: Corneal complications from herpes zoster ophthalmicus. *Ophthalmology* 1985; 92:316–324.
2. Marguiles LJ, Mannis MJ: Dendritic corneal lesions associated with soft contact lens wear. *Arch Ophthalmol* 1983; 101:1551–1553.
3. Seedor JA, Waring GO III: Dendriform lesions of the cornea induced by soft contact lenses. *Arch Ophthalmol* 1987; 105:1021.
4. Darougar S, Wishart MS, Viswalinggam ND: Epidemiological and clinical features of primary herpes simplex virus ocular infection. *Br J Ophthalmol* 1985; 69:2–6.
5. Parlato CJ, Cohen EJ, Sakauye CM, et al: Role of debridement and trifluridine (trifluorothymidine) in herpes simplex dendritic keratitis. *Arch Ophthalmol* 1985; 103:673–675.
6. Wittpenn JR Jr, Pepose JS, Dunkel EC, et al: Impression debridement for herpes simplex dendritic keratitis. *Ophthalmology* 1986; 93(suppl):114.
7. Schwab IR, Raju VK, McClung J: Indirect immunofluorescent antibody diagnosis of herpes simplex with upper tarsal and corneal scrapings. *Ophthalmology* 1986; 93:752–756.
8. Epstein RJ, Wilson LA, Visvesvara GS, et al: Rapid diagnosis of *Acanthamoeba* keratitis from corneal scrapings using indirect fluorescent antibody staining. *Arch Ophthalmol* 1986; 104:1318–1321.
9. McGill J: The enigma of herpes stromal disease. *Br J Ophthalmol* 1987; 71:118–125.
10. McNeill JI, Kaufman HE: Local antivirals in a herpes simplex stromal keratitis model. *Arch Ophthalmol* 1979; 97:727–729.
11. Kaufman HE, Centifanto-Fitzgerald YM, Varnell ED: Herpes simplex keratitis. *Ophthalmology* 1983; 90:700–706.

Approach 2

Kirk R. Wilhelmus, M.D.

This patient presents with a dendritic corneal ulcer that may well be the first clinical manifestation of herpes simplex eye disease in this individual. Generally, a clinical diagnosis can be substantiated by slit-lamp biomicroscopy alone, although new laboratory tests are becoming available for rapid diagnostic confirmation.

Clinical Diagnosis

Herpes simplex epithelial keratitis in an adult is almost always a manifestation of recurrent disease. Nevertheless, primary blepharoconjunctivitis should always be excluded by noting the absence of cutaneous and lid margin vesicles or unilateral follicular conjunctivitis. Adult men are affected more often than women, but frequently a triggering factor is not readily apparent.

Typical clinical features of dendritic keratitis are localized punctate epithelial keratitis lesions that coalesce to form an arborizing pattern, subsequently giving rise to a linear ulceration by autolysis of infected cells. Rose bengal 1% eyedrops are especially helpful to selectively stain swollen epithelial cells along the edge of the ulcerated lesion to highlight the branching dendrite with its terminal bulbs.

A few corneal conditions may occasionally simulate herpes simplex dendritic keratitis such as epithelial regeneration lines, epithelial basement membrane dystrophy, contact lens–associated keratopathy, thimerosal toxicity and other chemical injuries, and coarse mucous plaques. Dendritiform corneal lesions may also occur during ophthalmic zoster infection and have rarely been noted early in the course of *Acanthamoeba* keratitis.

Laboratory Evaluation

Because of the nearly pathognomonic clinical features of herpes simplex epithelial keratitis, laboratory testing is not usually necessary in routine clinical practice. Serological testing of blood samples is generally positive in most adults because of prior infection, although an absence of detectable antibody can help to exclude herpes simplex virus as a cause of atypical keratitis. Conjunctival scrapings and swabbings have been used for diagnostic testing but are frequently of low yield. A corneal debridement specimen is the most satisfactory way for confirming the diagnosis of herpes simplex epithelial keratitis.

The corneal sample may be smeared onto a glass slide and, after fixation, processed for Papanicolaou staining to reveal typical Cowdry type A eosinophilic intranuclear inclusions. Material can also be obtained for electron microscopy and viral culture, although frequently these are not readily available or are costly. For isolation, a cotton-tipped applicator rather than a calcium alginate one can be used to directly inoculate viral transport medium to be immediately sent on ice to the tissue cell culture laboratory.

Of greater potential clinical use is the recent availability of several rapid diagnostic tests for herpes simplex virus. Pilot studies have been done with an immunofluorescent assay, MicroTrak (Syva, Palo Alto, Calif), in which the corneal debridement specimen is smeared onto a glass slide, stained with fluoresceinated antiherpes antibody, and then examined with immunofluorescent microscopy. Rapid confirmation can be obtained in less than 1 hour. Other immunofluorescent assays (CultureSet, Ortho Diagnostics, Raritan, NJ; Virgo Antigen Detection System, Electro-Nucleonics, Columbia, Md) are becoming available as well as enzyme immunoassays and DNA probes (such as the HSV Patho-Gene Kit, Enzo Biochem, New York). The use of these rapid diagnostic techniques remains to be determined for clinical ophthalmologists.

Value of Debridement

Corneal epithelial debridement not only provides material for diagnostic laboratory evaluation but also is an adjuvant mechanical treatment for herpes simplex epithelial keratitis. Methods such as chemical cauterization can result in corneal scarring and have generally been abandoned. However, minimal wiping debridement is generally nondamaging and fairly precise.

In this technique, a topical anesthetic agent is applied (along with rose bengal eyedrops), and a sterile cotton-tipped applicator is wiped or rolled across the area of active infection to remove the virus-infected cells of the ulcer margins. Sharp dissection with a spatula is also effective but has a greater potential for producing inadvertent scarring. Wiping debridement is easy to perform, probably because the disrupted intercellular bridges of infected epithelium reduces cellular adherence. Because small focal punctate epithelial keratitis lesions may recur following debridement, supplemental antiviral therapy should then be begun. (Because of the potential teratogenic effects of some antiviral agents, debridement may provide the only necessary therapy for pregnant women.)

The principal benefit of mechanical debridement is the reduction in healing time with faster re-epithelialization. Several clinical trials have substantiated this advantage (Table 7–1), although others have failed to do so. Because recovery may be speeded by only 1 to 2 days, daily follow-up is necessary in order to detect the clinical effect. In addition, trials that have shown a beneficial effect of debridement have generally begun topical antiviral therapy immediately rather than delaying initiation of treatment to the following morning.

Epithelial healing re-establishes a protective ocular surface barrier and reduces symptoms, thereby enabling the patient to minimize lost workdays. A shorter healing time has also been suggested to reduce the recurrence rate.

Some additional theoretical advantages for debridement include removing the epithelial barrier to promote better corneal penetration of the antiviral agent. Debridement could also potentially reduce the subepithelial "ghost" opacity that sometimes follows dendritic keratitis. In addition, if the virus load of the corneal surface is removed, subsequent stromal inflammation could be minimized. However, these potential effects have not yet been substantiated.

TABLE 7–1.

Selected Clinical Trials Assessing the Value of Debridement With Topical Antiviral Therapy for Dendritic Keratitis

Source, yr	Trial Design	Antiviral Agent	Debridement Speeds Healing?
Whitcher et al., 1976	Uncontrolled	Idoxuridine	Yes
Egerer, 1979	Uncontrolled	Vidarabine	Yes
Herbort et al., 1985	Uncontrolled	Trifluridine	Yes
Wilhelmus et al., 1981	Controlled	Acyclovir	Yes
Jensen et al., 1982	Controlled	Acyclovir	No
Parlato et al., 1985	Controlled	Trifluridine	No
Herbort et al., 1987	Controlled	Trifluridine	Yes
Shimomura et al., 1987	Controlled	Idoxuridine	No

The limitations of debridement include the need for a cooperative patient, thereby limiting its use in children, and the risk of injury to the epithelial basement membrane and Bowman's layer. Thus, debridement is usually not utilized in large geographic keratitis lesions.

Antiviral Selection

Since the introduction of ophthalmic antiviral chemotherapy 25 years ago, several antiviral compounds have been investigated. Three agents, idoxuridine, vidarabine, and trifluridine, are now commercially available in the United States as topical preparations for herpes simplex epithelial keratitis. The choice of an antiviral drug should be based upon its pharmacological advantages, its cost and availability, and the patient's history of previous adverse reactions. All of the available agents are effective in the treatment of dendritic keratitis (Table 7–2), although trifluridine has been favored by some.

An optimal treatment of this business executive with dendritic keratitis would be minimal wiping debridement with the immediate institution of trifluridine 1% eyedrops 5 to 8 times per day. Idoxuridine and vidarabine remain effective alternative agents to be used should active epithelial keratitis persist with trifluridine therapy beyond 7 to 10 days or if an adverse reaction occurs. These agents are also available as ointments and may be preferable for young children because of ease of application.

Unfortunately, there is no evidence that the choice of the initial topical antiviral therapy or the use of debridement can reduce the risk of recurrent epithelial keratitis. The safety and efficacy of oral acyclovir in the treatment of herpetic keratitis and in the prevention of recurrences are currently under investigation.

Summary

Effective therapy for recurrent herpes simplex epithelial keratitis includes the combination of minimal wiping debridement and antiviral therapy to remove the virus-laden epithelial cells and to halt viral replication.

This patient may best be treated with minimal wiping debridement and immediate initiation of antiviral chemotherapy with trifluridine solution along with a cycloplegic eyedrop. Follow-up evaluations would continue until after re-epithelialization is completed. He should understand the nature of herpetic eye disease

TABLE 7–2.

Selected Clinical Trials Comparing Topical Antiviral Agents Currently Available in the United States for Dendritic Keratitis

Source, yr	Idoxuridine	Vidarabine	Trifluridine
Pavan-Langston et al., 1972	+*	+	
Hyndiuk et al., 1975	+	+	
Laibson et al., 1975	+	+	
Pavan-Langston et al., 1975	+	+	
Blake et al., 1977	+	+	
Markham et al., 1977	+	+	
Chin et al., 1978	+	+	
McKinnon et al., 1975		+	+
Travers et al., 1976		+	+
van Bijsterveld et al., 1980		+	+
Welling et al., 1972	+		+ +
Laibson et al., 1977	+		+
Pavan-Langston et al., 1977	+		+ +
Sugar et al., 1980	+		+

*+, Effective; + +, significantly more effective.

and know that he may have a fifty-fifty chance of another "attack" in the next few years or could develop visually disabling stromal keratitis.

Bibliography

1. Coster DJ, Jones BR, Falcon MG: Role of debridement in the treatment of herpetic keratitis. *Trans Ophthalmol Soc UK* 1977; 97:314–317.
2. Wilhelmus KR, Coster DJ, Donovan HC, et al: Prognostic indicators of herpetic keratitis. Analysis of a five-year observation period after corneal ulceration. *Arch Ophthalmol* 1981; 99:1578–1582.

SECTION III

Glaucoma

Glaucoma—Drops, Laser, or Surgery?

APPROACH 1

Thom J. Zimmerman, M.D., Ph.D.
David Linn, M.D.

APPROACH 2

Thomas A. Deutsch, M.D.

Case 8 _____

Glaucoma—Drops, Laser, or Surgery?

A 62-year-old man is found during a routine examination to have an intraocular pressure (IOP) of 35 mm Hg in the right eye and 39 mm Hg in the left. The right visual field has moderate inferior-nasal loss, and the left visual field has extensive nasal loss encroaching on fixation. The cup-to-disc ratio is 0.7 in the right eye and 0.9 in the left.

What is the appropriate treatment at this point?

Summary

When making a diagnosis of advanced glaucoma, the clinician is confronted with the need to lower the IOP sufficiently to prevent any further visual field loss. Should this be done with medications or surgery?

In their discussion, Drs. Zimmerman and Linn point out that most patients can be controlled with medical therapy. They advocate starting with several topical medications and then backing off to the minimal medicines necessary to keep the IOP under 20 mm Hg.

In my approach, I stress that the IOP is but one aspect of the evaluation of glaucoma "control" while assessment of changes in the visual field is more important in advanced cases. In the case of this patient's left eye, any change in the field that signifies inadequate control could signal loss of fixation and hence useful vision. Therefore, I advocate an aggressive approach using filtering surgery in the left eye.

Both of the discussions of this case emphasize the importance of evaluating the visual fields again in 3 to 4 months. In the initial evaluation of glaucoma it is tempting to become so involved in "controlling" the IOP that the goal of therapy—preservation of vision—is forgotten.

Approach 1

Thom J. Zimmerman, M.D., Ph.D.
David Linn, M.D.

A 62-year-old white male was found with IOPs of 35 mm Hg OD and 39 mm Hg OS, significant visual field changes, and cup-to-disc ratios of 0.7 OD and 0.9 OS. The question is, "What is the appropriate treatment?"

The overall approach to a new patient workup would begin with a complete history including age, sex, race, family histories, general medical history, past ocular histories, traumas, and all ocular and systemic medications. In addition, any past ocular examinations, visual field testings, etc., should be queried. A complete eye exam would include visual acuity, manifest refraction, external examination, slit-lamp examination, IOPs, gonioscopy, funduscopic examination, stereo disc photos, and automated static visual fields.

Assuming this patient has chronic open-angle glaucoma, i.e., no previous evidence of eye surgery or trauma, first detections of elevated IOPs, and normal angles, usually one would start with a β-blocker, timolol (Timoptic) (0.25%), one drop twice daily unless contraindicated by medical history. We have recently shown that 0.25% Timoptic is at the top of the dose-response curve. One would discuss with the patient the proper technique for using eye drops. This would include nasolacrimal occlusion and gentle eyelid closure for 3 to 5 minutes, with additional drops spaced at least 10 minutes apart and the patient reclining to allow maximum contact of the drug to the eye. If the patient had a contraindication to Timoptic, i.e., asthma, perhaps the substitution of betaxolol (Betoptic) would be suitable. One must remember that the difference between a nonselective β-blocker such as Timoptic or levobunolol (Betagan) and a selective β-blocker like Betoptic is relative and not absolute. A patient who would respond adversely to a nonselective β-blocker may respond similarly to the current selective one. One can always do monocular trials to conclude whether indeed a patient is a drug responder and to assess the side effects at half the dose. If additional drugs are necessary, we would add a miotic—for this white male, 2% pilocarpine twice daily. We have recently shown that 2% pilocarpine twice daily gives a maximum effect for a full 24 hours. We recommend the use of 2% pilocarpine 10 minutes following the Timoptic. Again, monocular testing can be performed to demonstrate the efficacy of the combination. Stronger miotics like carbachol in a twice daily dosing have also been found to be quite efficacious following a β-blocker or epinephrine. Our experience with Propine or epinephrine in conjunction with Timoptic has not usually been found to be useful: only one of five patients will have a significant long-term additivity. We therefore go from a β-blocker to a miotic of some type and then to a carbonic anhydrase inhibitor as a third step. Methazolamide, 25 mg twice daily, would be a reasonable starting point. Methazolamide, 50 mg twice daily is a maximal dose and has a higher frequency of side effects. One can change the patient's therapy from methazolamide, 50 mg twice daily to acetazolamide, 500-mg sequels twice daily and perhaps get increased efficacy.

In this particular patient with presumed optic nerve damage and corresponding visual field changes, it would be appropriate to start aggressively with topical medicines (0.25% Timoptic and 2% pilocarpine) for quicker control and then back down to the minimal medicines needed to stop the advance of disease. The goals of treatment for this patient would be an IOP of less than 20 with continuing proof of stabilization of the discs and visual fields. If adequate IOPs were obtained with medical therapy, one would do repeat automated static perimetry and disc examination every 3 to 4 months to assess efficacy.

If indeed this approach was not successful and/or tolerance or compliance were major problems, then doing a 180-degree argon laser trabeculoplasty with 50-μm spots at the appropriate power settings to get blanching of the anterior trabecular meshwork would be the next step. Treatment with the other 180 degrees would follow if control was still inadequate. If control was still not obtained, then surgical intervention would be indicated.

Approach 2

Thomas A. Deutsch, M.D.

Briefly stated, this case concerns a 62-year-old man with newly diagnosed glaucoma. The IOP is quite high, and there is moderate visual field loss in the right eye and extensive loss in the left eye.

The classic approach to the management of glaucoma involves initiation of treatment with eyedrops and addition of a carbonic anhydrase inhibitor if the IOP remains uncontrolled. Laser trabeculoplasty is done next if the pressure is still too high, with filtering surgery as a last resort. The rationale for this approach is that most patients will respond to medications with sufficient lowering of the IOP to avoid laser or filtering surgery. However, I would argue that the extensive visual field loss in this case mandates a more aggressive approach if vision is to be retained.

It is important to discuss the definition of the term *control* in the context of glaucoma management. IOP is one measure of control, but since we do not know what the optimal pressure is for any given eye, it can only be used as a guide to the relative efficacy of treatment. Far more important is the evaluation of the way in which the field is responding to therapy. In other words, no matter what the IOP is, if the visual field worsens, then the pressure must be lowered. Dependence on the *number* alone will lead the clinician astray. This is especially true when the optic nerve is already greatly compromised, as in this case, since such a nerve may be even more susceptible to the pressure than would a normal eye.

In the case described here, we cannot afford to wait and find out whether any pressure will be tolerated, i.e., will prevent further field loss. Any further field loss in the left eye will result in blindness! In the left eye, IOP must be lowered quickly and definitively.

Luckily, the right eye is not as severely affected as the left, so there is time to give the right eye medical therapy and possibly do a laser treatment while the left eye recovers from filtering surgery. The management of the right eye is complicated by the fact that some of the medicine directed at that eye will also affect the left and cause decreased aqueous production and compromise development of the filtering bleb. β-Blockers are well known to provide a contralateral effect, and carbonic anhydrase inhibitors obviously will affect both eyes. Thus, the maximal medications that can be used in the right eye are a miotic and an epinephrine product. It is unlikely that these will be sufficient to lower the pressure to a safe level, and so laser trabeculoplasty will probably be necessary.

My specific recommendations for the right eye are to administer 2% pilocarpine and Propine. Unless the pressure fell below 20 with this therapy, I would proceed with a laser trabeculoplasty. In either case, the visual field examination should be repeated in 3 months to detect any progression. I would schedule a trabeculectomy in the left eye at the earliest opportunity.

Now, why not start with laser trabeculoplasty in the left eye as well? First, as stated earlier, we are not in any position to wait and see whether laser therapy provides sufficient pressure lowering to prevent further field loss. Second, postlaser IOP spikes, a well-reported phenomenon, could result in loss of fixation. It is far more prudent to aim for maximal pressure lowering immediately and save the remaining visual field.

Cataract and Glaucoma—To Filter or Not to Filter?

APPROACH 1

Marianne E. Feitl, M.D.
Theodore Krupin, M.D.

APPROACH 2

Jon M. Ruderman, M.D.

Case 9 _____

Cataract and Glaucoma—To Filter or Not to Filter?

A 62-year-old woman has been under glaucoma treatment for many years. She is currently using timolol, pilocarpine, and epinephrine in each eye and acetazolamide. Laser trabeculoplasty has been performed in each eye. The intraocular pressures are 20 in the right eye and 18 in the left. Her right eye has developed a cataract that reduces the visual acuity to 20/100. The visual acuity in the left eye is 20/40 with nuclear sclerotic lens changes.

The patient wants an improvement in her visual acuity but is concerned about her glaucoma control. What is the best approach to her management?

Summary _____

This patient has borderline-controlled intraocular pressure with maximal medication and an operable cataract. In this day of microsurgery it is technically possible to perform combined cataract and filtration surgery, but the question is whether this technical ability translates into a benefit to the patient.

Doctors Feitl and Krupin present the case for cataract surgery alone. They point out that, although there have really been no controlled trials, several studies have demonstrated that many (if not most) glaucomatous eyes will maintain good intraocular pressure control after extracapsular cataract extraction (ECCE) with posterior-chamber intraocular lens (PC-IOL) implantation. The catch is that the pressure should be "controlled" prior to surgery, a condition only barely present in this case.

In outlining his approach, Dr. Ruderman goes over both the complications of combined surgery and the indications. A patient with advanced optic nerve damage is at risk of losing central vision following cataract surgery in the immediate postoperative period. Therefore, a combined procedure using a tightly sutured trabeculectomy flap may blunt the common postoperative intraocular pressure rise that is often seen after cataract extraction alone.

Cataract surgery in the glaucomatous eye is trickier and fraught with more complications than in the nonglaucomatous eye. The possible need for iris manipulation, care of the conjunctiva, astigmatism, and postoperative visual rehabilitation of an eye with field loss are among the problems. All of these experts agree that, where possible, the patient will be better served by separate procedures to treat the cataract and the glaucoma.

Approach 1 _____

Marianne E. Feitl, M.D.
Theodore Krupin, M.D.

We believe that the surgical management of a glaucoma patient with a visually handicapping cataract must be based on the patient's glaucoma control. Adequate intraocular pressure for a given patient is determined on an individual basis. This patient's intraocular pressure, 20 mm Hg, falls into a borderline zone. If she has had a stable visual field and an unchanged cup-to-disc ratio at this level of intraocular pressure, we would consider her to be under adequate glaucoma medical control. We are making the assumption that she is tolerating her medications without ocular or systemic side effects. Given a background of good intraocular pressure control and a significant cataract that is reducing vision, our primary concern is how to best improve her vision without subjecting her to undue risks or a reduction in the level of her glaucoma control.

Several approaches to cataract extraction in glaucoma patients are possible. If the patient's intraocular pressure is poorly controlled with maximum medical therapy, a combined cataract extraction and filtration operation may be warranted. A combined procedure may also be indicated in patients with controlled intraocular pressures but poor tolerance to their medical therapy or in patients with controlled pressures but extensive visual field loss in which the ophthalmologist feels an even lower intraocular pressure is needed. Combined surgery does have a higher risk of postoperative complications, however, including a flat anterior chamber, hyphema, prolonged postoperative hypotony, and choroidal detachment. Also, visual recovery may be more prolonged. Thus, unless the patient requires a filtration procedure for glaucoma control, we feel it is best to proceed with only the lower-risk cataract procedure. ECCE with PC-IOL implantation alone may be the best choice in these patients for restoring vision and maintaining intraocular pressure control.

In the past, studies have shown that *intracapsular* cataract extraction in patients with glaucoma was associated with stable or improved postoperative intraocular pressure control with the same or fewer medications.[1] Currently, ECCE with PC-IOL is the most commonly applied technique in the United States for cataract removal. Several authors have demonstrated that ECCE with PC-IOL in glaucomatous eyes does not have an adverse effect on postoperative intraocular pressure levels.[2-6] Recent studies have found that intraocular pressure control is improved in about 57% to 70% of patients, unchanged in 16% to 41% of patients, and made worse in only 2% to 9% of patients.[4, 6] Another group reported achieving a postoperative intraocular pressure below 21 mm Hg in 50% of eyes with the same number of medications as used before the cataract surgery, 25% with fewer medications, and 25% with more medications than used preoperatively.[5]

The placement of a PC-IOL avoids potential trabecular damage by the lens haptics, which is a concern with anterior chamber lenses. Anterior chamber IOLs may damage the trabecular meshwork and further compromise aqueous outflow by inducing peripheral anterior synechiae, by inducing a low-grade trabeculitis, and by vascular proliferation around the haptics in the anterior-chamber angle. Additionally, in the event that filtration surgery becomes necessary, posterior chamber lenses have less risk of corneal endothelial contact should a shallow or flat anterior chamber occur. We do not use anterior chamber implants in eyes with glaucoma.

Although long-term intraocular pressure control is generally stable following ECCE with PC-IOL in glaucoma patients, substantial increases in intraocular pressure have been noted in the early postoperative period. Increases in intraocular pressure can also occur following similar cataract surgery in the nonglaucoma patient. We have observed postoperative pressure elevations even when a combined filtering procedure and cataract extraction has been performed. Glaucoma patients have a much higher incidence of early postoperative pressure rises than do normal patients.[3, 5] Posterior chamber lens implantation does not increase the occurrence of this complication. The glaucomatous eye has a compromised outflow system and, thus, is less able to deal with obstructive substances incurred during cataract surgery. Cataract extraction alone, without the use of viscoelastic material, can cause a short-term pressure elevation. Viscoelastic material in the anterior chamber has been shown to decrease outflow facility in eyes at autopsy.[7] Cortical material, viscoelastic substances, red blood cells, pigmented iris cells, and inflammatory cells may all contribute to this effect. Since preoperative miotic glaucoma therapy is common, pupillary dilation may be poor in these patients. Therefore, additional iris manipulation with pigment and inflammatory cell release can be expected. Special attention must therefore be given to the potential development of a pressure rise in the early postoperative period in these patients.

Cataract extraction may result in improved postoperative medical management of the glaucoma patient. In addition, miotics may be poorly tolerated in the glaucoma patient with a cataract. However, these agents are effective and well tolerated in the aphakic eye. Also, phospholine iodide is well tolerated and very effective in aphakic and pseudophakic patients. Conversely, additional caution is necessary with the use of epinephrine compounds due to the risk of aphakic cystoid macular edema.[8] This epinephrine-induced complication, which can also occur following dipivalyl epinephrine (Propine) use, has a reported incidence between 10% to 20%. However, epinephrine cystoid macular edema is reversible when treatment with the medication is discontinued. We use epinephrine therapy in the aphakic glaucoma patient with careful monitoring of the visual acuity and the appearance of the macula.

Cataract surgery, in particular ECCE with PC-IOL, is more complicated in the glaucoma patient. Miotic therapy limits pupillary dilation, and posterior synechiae may be present. We perform a peripheral iridectomy in all glaucoma eyes. After viscoelastic material is instilled into the anterior chamber, the synechiae should be swept with a cyclodialysis spatula placed through the iridectomy and through the pupil. If pupillary dilation is poor, inferior sphincterotomies may be made to allow adequate space for nucleus removal and posterior-chamber lens implantation.

When this does not allow sufficient space, the peripheral iridectomy can be converted to a sector iridectomy. Additional viscoelastic material may aid in exposure during the capsulotomy by displacing and holding the iris leaflets away from the cataract. It is important to remove as much viscoelastic material as possible at the end of surgery to minimize its effect on pressure elevation.

If a sector iridectomy is performed, it need not be sutured closed. The additional surgical manipulation may increase the risk of hemorrhage or corneal problems. Patients do not generally complain of visual symptoms from a sector iridectomy. Additionally, disc observation may be facilitated through the iridectomy, particularly in those patients who require continued miotics.

In the early postoperative period, intraocular pressure must be carefully monitored and antiglaucoma therapy continued. Pilocarpine administration may be suspended temporarily since this agent can increase postoperative inflammation. Steroid drops should be used as needed to control inflammation. Caution is advised in the use of long-acting subconjunctivival steroid injections because of the potential steroid-induced pressure rise in the glaucomatous eye. Similarly, the long-term use of topical steroid drops must be carefully monitored for this effect. Steroid therapy should be tapered and discontinued as soon as possible.

A new baseline visual field and optic disc evaluation should be undertaken as soon as possible. The visual fields may improve after cataract extraction, and further comparisons should be made against the postoperative field. Also, detailed visualization and photography of the optic disc may be possible at this time.

Although most glaucoma patients do well with medical therapy after ECCE with PC-IOL, a small number of patients may develop uncontrolled intraocular pressure and progressive visual field damage. Argon laser trabeculoplasty is successful in 50% to 60% of pseudophakic eyes.[9] However, we would not repeat laser therapy if it had already been performed, as is the situation in the patient under discussion. Finally, if still indicated, we would perform a filtration procedure.

The long-term success rate for filtration surgery performed either as combined surgery with a posterior-chamber lens implant or separately at a later time following cataract removal is unreported. Further studies and long-term follow-up are needed to obtain this information. As surgical techniques and materials are modified, continued evaluation will be required to determine the best approach to the glaucoma patient requiring cataract surgery.

References

1. Bigger JF, Becker B: Cataracts and primary open-angle glaucoma: The effect of uncomplicated cataract extraction on glaucoma control. *Ophthalmology* 1971; 75:260.
2. Radius RL, Schultz K, Sobocinski K, et al: Pseudophakia and intraocular pressure. *Am J Ophthalmol* 1984; 97:738.
3. Savage JA, Thomas JV, Belcher CD, et al: Extracapsular cataract extraction and posterior chamber intraocular lens implantation in glaucomatous eyes. *Ophthalmology* 1985; 92:1506.
4. McMahan LB, Monica ML, Zimmerman TJ: Posterior chamber pseudophakes in glaucoma patients. *Ophthalmic Surg* 1986; 17:146.
5. McGuigan LJB, Gottsch J, Stark WJ, et al: Extracapsular cataract extraction and posterior chamber lens implantation in eyes with preexisting glaucoma. *Arch Ophthalmol* 1986; 104:1301.
6. Handa J, Henry JC, Krupin T, et al: Extracapsular cataract extraction with posterior chamber lens implantation in patients with glaucoma. *Arch Ophthalmol* 1987; 105:765.
7. Berson FG, Patterson MM, Epstein DL: Obstruction of aqueous outflow by sodium hyaluronate in enucleated human eyes. *Am J Ophthalmol* 1983; 95:668.
8. Kolker AE, Becker B: Epinephrine maculopathy. *Arch Ophthalmol* 1968; 79:552.
9. Krupin T: Anterior segment laser surgery, in Krupin T, Waltman SR (eds): *Complications in Ophthalmic Surgery*, ed 2. Philadelphia, JB Lippincott, 1984, pp 175–192.

Approach 2

Jon M. Ruderman, M.D.

Determination of a "best approach" to the problem of combined glaucoma and cataract depends on a number of factors that were not addressed in the history. Those questions that need to be answered include

- How severe is the glaucoma?
- Has there been optic nerve damage?
- What is the status of the visual field?
- Does the patient's vision improve when the pupil is dilated?
- Is the patient compliant with medical therapy?
- How disabled is the patient with her current vision?
- Would the patient accept more than one operation?
- Is the patient a potential contact lens candidate?
- Has she ever had ocular inflammation or prior conjunctival surgery?
- Does she have open-angle glaucoma or angle-closure glaucoma?

Medical and Surgical Management

A basic principle in managing a patient with both cataract and glaucoma is to control or treat the glaucoma first. Uncontrolled glaucoma in an aphakic or pseudophakic patient is more difficult to treat than is uncontrolled glaucoma in a phakic individual. In my opinion, simultaneous surgery for both the glaucoma and cataract should be undertaken only when there is a definite indication for both procedures and the patient is not willing or able to undergo two procedures.

Major problems with simultaneous filtration and cataract surgery are inevitable since the goals of these operations are dissimilar. A cataract operation is designed for visual rehabilitation. This is best achieved by meticulous and complete wound closure. The goal of a glaucoma procedure, however, is to create a permanent leak from the anterior chamber into a subconjunctival filtration bleb. A wound defect created to establish filtration increases the complication rate in a patient who undergoes simultaneous cataract surgery. After a combined procedure the intraocular pressure usually stays very low for the first few postoperative weeks. Blood vessels in the wound that were not cauterized at the time of surgery may bleed. The resulting hyphema and blood breakdown products can contribute toward failure of the filtration procedure. Inflammation caused by extensive surgery on the anterior segment (especially on an iris made rigid by years of miotic therapy) may also increase inflammation and lead to a greater incidence of filtration failure. In addition, postoperative astigmatism is greater in combined procedures and controlling this by cutting sutures is difficult because of the presence of a filtration bleb.

With the preceding in mind, there are some situations that call for combined surgery. A patient may require both a cataract extraction and a filtration procedure but will not accept or be physically able to tolerate two separate operations. If the patient needs immediate visual rehabilitation (e.g., if there is a dense cataract in both eyes), then combined surgery may be indicated. A combined procedure may be the treatment of choice if a patient lives far from the physicians' office and might not be able to complete the follow-up visits that multiple surgeries would entail.

A scheme for management of combined cataract and glaucoma is summarized in Fig 9–1. If the patient's glaucoma is under control, the patient is compliant, and the optic nerve is not significantly damaged, then cataract surgery alone will probably be sufficient. Most reports suggest that open-angle glaucoma is neither improved nor made worse by cataract surgery. If, on the other hand, the glaucoma is severe (either the intraocular pressure is uncontrolled or the optic nerve is severely damaged), then a filtering operation is indicated first.

In some instances a cataract extraction with a "tight" trabeculectomy filtration procedure is indicated. For instance, a patient may have a cataract and a low intraocular pressure but have evidence of severe optic nerve damage that occurred years previously. This type of patient might be cared for by cataract extraction and implantation of a posterior chamber lens. However, in this age of tight wound closure, sodium hyaluronate, and extracapsular lens extraction, postoperative elevations of intraocular pressure to extremely high levels (50 to 60 mm Hg) are not uncommon because of the compromised outflow pathway in the eye. A healthy optic nerve is able to handle a pressure of 50 mm Hg for 1 to 5 days. A previously damaged optic nerve in the same situation may sustain enough additional damage to produce severe visual loss. A combined procedure with a tight trabeculectomy flap has been helpful in eliminating severe postoperative intraocular pressure elevations while still giving reasonable control over the cataract wound.

There are other considerations when making a decision in patients with cataract and glaucoma. Is the patient going to require a contact lens at some point in the future? If this is the case, a cyclodialysis may be the best treatment, although it has been associated with a high incidence of intraocular hemorrhage in the past. If the patient has had prior surgery on the eye and the conjunctiva is scarred, then a cataract extraction, posterior-chamber lens implantation, and cyclodialysis may be the best form of therapy. Alternatively, a drug that alters wound healing, such as 5-fluorouracil may make it possible to perform a filter on a patient with conjunctival scarring.

If the patient has angle-closure glaucoma, then a laser iridot-

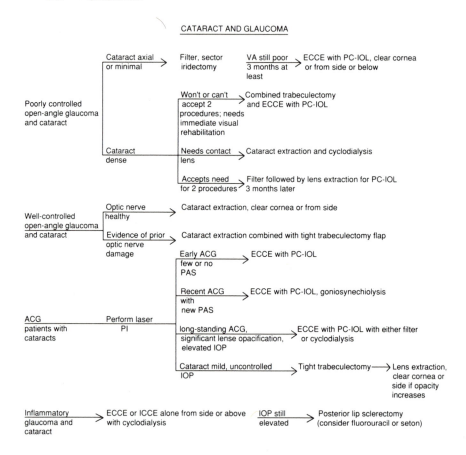

FIG 9–1.
Scheme for management of combined cataract and glaucoma. PI = peripheral iridotomy.

omy is indicated prior to any procedure. If the angle widens and the intraocular pressure is controlled following laser iridotomy, then a simple cataract extraction should be sufficient to keep the glaucoma under control. If the angle closure is of recent onset, then a cataract extraction combined with synechiolysis (a procedure in which a cyclodialysis spatula is used to separate peripheral anterior synechiae from the trabecular meshwork) may be employed. Frequently, an iridotomy is performed and the intraocular pressure is still elevated. In this case the density of the cataract is crucial. A filtration procedure performed with a sector iridectomy and tight scleral flap in order to avoid a flat anterior chamber is indicated if the cataract is not very dense. If the cataract is mature, a combined procedure is indicated.

When a simple cataract procedure is performed in a patient with glaucoma, the decision must be made as to where to place the incision. Aphakic filters fail primarily because the conjunctiva has had previous surgery. If a surgical procedure for glaucoma might be needed following a cataract extraction, then it is wise to leave some "virgin" conjunctiva superonasally. A cataract can be taken out by using a superotemporal or side approach.

Combined Cataract Extraction and Filtration Procedure Technique

Patients who are candidates for a combined procedure should be informed that it will take longer for them to regain their vision than for most patients who undergo cataract surgery. They also must be informed of the increased risk of complications, especially hemorrhage, astigmatism, and wound leak. After a standard preparation and draping, a 4-0 silk superior rectus suture is placed as far posteriorly as possible in the fornix, and the eye is rotated downward. A fornix-based flap is fashioned from 9 to 3 o'clock. It is necessary to adequately free up the conjunctiva from the underlying scleral surface so that it can be brought down tightly over the superior wound at the end of the procedure. After adequate hemostasis is achieved, a 64 Beaver blade is used to create a scleral groove at the posterior margin of the limbus until 12:30. At that point a triangular flap 5 mm long along the base and 5 mm in height is fashioned. The flap should be about a one-half scleral thickness. The remainder of the scleral groove is completed on the other side of the triangular flap. A paracentesis tract that will be used to test the rate of filtration and the tightness of the conjunctival wound is fashioned. The anterior chamber is entered to the side of the triangular flap with a Superblade. Sodium hyaluronate is instilled in the eye, and an anterior capsulotomy using a bent 25-gauge needle is performed. If the pupil is small, a radial iridectomy, lysis of iridocapsular adhesions, and a sphinctero-tomy are all performed. After the capsulotomy the nucleus is loos-ened, and the corneoscleral wound is opened. Care is taken to avoid cutting the scleral flap. The nucleus is prolapsed out of the eye by using a muscle hook and a .12 forceps to create some countertraction. Alternatively a lens loop with a serrated edge can be used to deliver the nucleus. Two 10-0 nylon sutures are placed on opposite sides of the scleral flap. After adequate irrigation and aspiration one of the side sutures is removed. Sodium hyaluronate is placed into the anterior chamber, and an IOL is placed in the capsular bag. The corneal wound is reapposed with 10-0 nylon sutures. A Kelly Descemet punch is used to remove two or three full-thickness pieces of the trabecular meshwork. The iris can then be repaired with a 10-0 Prolene suture either by prolapsing it or by using a straight 20-gauge needle. In most patients with severe field loss, this closure is strictly cosmetic. Subsequently, the scleral flap is sewn at the top (and sides if necessary) to decrease the rate of fluid egress from the anterior chamber. Fluid is next instilled into the anterior chamber through the paracentesis tract to see whether the sclerectomy is filtering. The conjunctiva is attached to the episcleral tissue at 9 and 3 o'clock with 9-0 Vicryl sutures. The wound is tested with 2% fluorescein, and 2 mg subconjunc-tival dexamethasone is given. Topical antibiotics and atropine are placed on the eye. A tight patch that may be removed the following day is applied. In the event that a wound leak appears along the edge of the filtration site, 10-0 nylon or 9-0 Vicryl sutures will effectively close the leak.

Increased Intraocular Pressure—Glaucoma Suspect or Glaucoma Patient?

APPROACH 1

Robert N. Weinreb, M.D.

APPROACH 2

Marc F. Lieberman, M.D.

Increased Intraocular Pressure— Glaucoma Suspect or Glaucoma Patient?

A 45-year-old man sees his ophthalmologist for refraction. Routine testing for glaucoma reveals an intraocular pressure (IOP) of 28 bilaterally. The cup-to-disc ratio is 0.3 in each eye, and computerized visual fields are normal. The patient's older brother is being followed for progressive visual field loss from glaucoma.

Should this patient be treated for glaucoma?

Summary

When does elevated IOP constitute glaucoma? The approach to this recurrent problem in clinical practice is the subject of this case discussion.

Our obligation to "do no harm" is the thrust of Dr. Weinreb's discussion. We should be cautious of starting treatment in patients who do not have glaucoma. Indeed, he points out that only about 1% of patients with elevated IOP will develop visual field loss. Interestingly, our ability to detect axonal loss from glaucoma with visual field testing is becoming more sophisticated all the time.

The importance of evaluating risk factors is emphasized by Dr. Lieberman in his discussion of this case. In addition to elevated IOP, the presence of progressive cupping, older age, and positive family history are among risk factors associated with visual field loss. Because of the positive family history of our patient, a trial of therapy, perhaps in one eye, seems indicated.

When informing patients of elevated IOP and discussing possible approaches, it is wise to admit our inability to separate glaucoma suspects from glaucoma patients. Both authors point out the importance of educating this patient about his condition and then adjusting therapy on the basis of his understanding and compliance.

Approach 1 _____

Robert N. Weinreb, M.D.

We are confronted with a 45-year-old man who has an IOP of 28 mm Hg in each eye. The cup disc ratio is 0.3 in each eye, and his computerized visual fields are normal. There is a family history of glaucoma, with an older brother who has had progressive visual field loss. The decision to initiate IOP-reducing therapy in a patient who is suspected of having glaucoma is often a difficult one. Although high IOP is associated with characteristic optic nerve atrophy and visual field loss, the maximum level of IOP that can be tolerated by an individual eye is not readily determined. The specific IOP level at which the optic nerve becomes damaged appears to vary among individuals. This variability is complicated by the difficulty in obtaining IOP data that reflect its changing levels throughout the day.

There are a number of reasons why one should not indiscriminately prescribe IOP-reducing medication to all patients with ocular hypertension. First and foremost is our increasing awareness of the potential of all topically administered drugs for having both ocular and systemic toxicity. The widespread use of topically administered β-blocking agents, for example, is associated with cardiovascular, pulmonary, and central nervous system effects that may cause or exacerbate disease. Our enthusiasm for reducing IOP in all eyes with high IOP is tempered also by the observation that most of these eyes have no evidence of optic nerve atrophy or visual field loss; when followed over several years, only approximately 1% of these eyes per year will develop visual field loss. Admittedly, it is possible that this rate is time dependent and that it might be higher than 1% per year after a considerable period of time. Unfortunately, long-term controlled studies testing this hypothesis are not available.

One argument that has been advanced in support of early treatment is based on the finding that a loss of optic nerve fibers precedes detectable visual field defects as characterized with the Goldmann perimeter. In these studies, one quarter to one third of the optic nerve fibers were atrophic without any change in the Goldmann visual field, and one half of the nerve was gone by the time a reproducible early paracentral scotoma or nasal step was detected. If these data can be confirmed in studies in which sensitive and reproducible automated perimetry is employed, the current rules governing our decision to initiate treatment in the glaucoma suspect would have to be modified.

Although the cup-to-disc ratio is 0.3, one should question whether this has changed compared with earlier examinations. Has there been progressive optic cup enlargement? Are there any peripapillary splinter hemorrhages or defects in the nerve fiber layer? Our ability to detect optic nerve damage and visual field loss is being refined with the introduction of new diagnostic techniques. Conventional methods of ophthalmoscopic examination have allowed us to recognize progressive optic cup enlargement, cup asymmetry, and peripapillary splinter hemorrhages as characteristic signs of optic nerve injury in many eyes. They may allow us to identify less characteristic changes including vertical cup elongation, undermining of cup edges, and prominent laminar pores throughout the cup. The possibility that defects in the nerve fiber layer can be used to predict which glaucoma suspects will develop visual field loss is also being evaluated. Most currently employed techniques only provide a subjective measure and, hence, have limited sensitivity for diagnosing glaucoma or recognizing its progression. New advances in instrumentation allow the topography of the optic disc and nerve fiber layer to be characterized objectively. Parameters such as neuroretinal rim area, cup volume, and surface topography are being investigated as predictive indicators of which eyes will develop glaucoma and require therapy.

Our ability to evaluate the function of the retina and optic nerve in glaucoma is also improving. Automated visual field testing provides standardized examinations with great accuracy and reproducibility. Many eyes with full Goldmann visual fields have been determined to have depressions in retinal threshold sensitivity at one or more locations with automated static testing. Either this represents an artifact with no consequence to the patient, or these changes indicate the detection of visual field loss earlier than previously possible. This can only be determined by following such eyes over a long period of time. Other tests of visual function are also being employed to diagnose glaucoma. The idea that central visual function is spared early in glaucoma is gradually being discarded. The measurement of Snellen visual acuity only measures the resolving power of the eye at near-maximum contrast and does not take into account such varied parameters as color vision, contrast perception, motion, and illumination. Tests that take them into account undoubtedly will contribute to our ability to distinguish those eyes that will ultimately be considered to have glaucoma from those that will not.

Having an older brother with glaucoma also raises our suspicion. Does our patient have myopia or pigmentary dispersion, both conditions having a greater chance of developing glaucoma? Our decision to treat is based on evidence of optic nerve damage or visual field loss in combination with risk factors that do not indicate damage but are associated with a greater likelihood that damage will occur. The older a patient, the more likely optic nerve damage will occur. Although the genetics of primary open-angle glaucoma is not well understood (polygenic multifactorial inheritance), there is no doubt that patients with a family history of glaucoma are at greater risk. The higher the IOP, the more likely an eye is to develop glaucoma. The larger the cup disc ratio, the greater the chance of visual field loss developing in an eye suspected of having glaucoma. Myopic individuals as well as those with pigmentary dispersion syndrome and pseudoexfoliation syndrome have a greater chance of developing glaucoma. This information is used to determine the likelihood that a patient will develop glaucoma.

We would propose withholding medical therapy in our patient until there is evidence of axonal or visual field loss. We would follow him to monitor the IOP at 3-month intervals and obtain visual field testing at least every 6 months. Stereoscopic images of the optic disc would facilitate subsequent evaluations. We would educate him about the significance of being diagnosed as a glaucoma suspect because of high IOP and family history. If he did not appear to be motivated to maintain our schedule of follow-up examinations, we might initiate therapy with either a β-blocking agent or an adrenergic agent. If the IOP consistently exceeded 30 mm Hg, we would consider giving the patient treatment as well. There is accumulating evidence that with such high pressures there is a greater probability of developing primary open-angle glaucoma.

Approach 2 _____

Marc F. Lieberman, M.D.

Much of the challenge of managing patients under suspicion for glaucoma is the mental calculus involved in deciding whether and how aggressively to treat a finding of elevated IOP. If we consider glaucoma as a spectrum, the "definite and unequivocal" wing includes the classic triad of elevated pressure plus damaged optic disc plus defective visual field. Management decisions in such circumstances are straightforward since the risks of the standard "staircase" approach—medications, then laser, then surgery—are felt to outweigh the risks of progressive glaucomatous disease. Should a pressure not come down, disc damage progress, or a field sprout a new or denser defect, then the next level of therapy is activated until clinical stability is achieved.

It's the other end of the glaucoma spectrum, where parts of the triad are "missing," that poses the difficult decisions. Such is this case of this young man with elevated pressures in both eyes but with apparently normal optic discs and fields. "Apparently normal" in this instance would mean that there is no evidence of the discs having changed from a smaller cup-to-disc ratio to their current 0.3 dimensions and that the computerized visual fields that were done involved full-threshold testing (and not just a screening examination) of the central 30 degrees.

Historical Risk Factors

This patient's situation is where the concept of "risk factors" comes into play. The clinician must assess whether there are a sufficient number of features, specific to the patient at hand, to warrant the initiation of therapy. At the same time, some thought should be given as to what features would justify either the escalation or the cessation of glaucoma therapy.

The first assessment of risk factors derives from the patient's family and personal history. Of great significance in this case is the fact that the patient's older brother is under care for "progressive visual field loss from glaucoma." This is very specific and helpful information; in obtaining a family history it is important to pinpoint details.* Further data about the brother's condition may have bearing in this case: at what age did the glaucoma begin? Were trauma or steroid use contributory? Are other factors such as diabetes or myopia involved? Besides a positive history for glaucoma among siblings, parents, or offspring, perhaps the next most useful piece of family history is whether there is diabetes mellitus among close relatives.

Similar questions about injury or steroid usage should be put to the patient himself. Sometimes steroid exposure per se is not recalled, but a history of long-standing asthma, eczema, or unusual arthritis will elicit the memory of prednisone use. Conversational inquiries into these matters can also reveal the quality of the patient's awareness of and concern for glaucoma. When the clinician appreciates aspects of the patient's psychological fabric such as a strong denial mechanism or undue anxiety, appropriate features of a therapeutic regimen and follow-up schedule can be designed.

Uncovering stories about prior ophthalmologic or optometric care can be particularly helpful, specifically if IOPs had high values in the past. The significance of the answer, though, is somewhat complex. In a large prospective series reported by Armaly, for example, nearly half of newly diagnosed glaucoma male patients had had normal pressure readings within 1 year of their field defects being detected; this suggests that a *change* in pressure status may be of prognostic significance.[1] On the other hand, many patients may tolerate a long-standing history of elevated pressures with no signs of developing disc and field loss and manifest a

---

*For example, a postcataract pressure rise after a grandmother's surgery may have been referred to as "glaucoma" but needed no further therapy, or a sister with a single measured pressure of 24 may be followed "for glaucoma" without evidence of true disease.

"resistance," as it were, to ocular hypertension.[2] If the patient indeed had been informed about his tonometry in the past, other historical documentation too, such as disc photographs, might be available.

Physical Risk Factors

The actual ophthalmic examination will reveal the presence of other risk factors known to correlate with bilateral glaucoma. Three findings most relevant in the age group of this 45-year-old patient would be the existence of myopia, of pigment dispersion stigmata, or of an anomalously appearing angle on gonioscopy.

There appears to be both a higher prevalence of glaucoma among myopes as well as a higher frequency of myopes among patients with open-angle glaucoma. This association holds even with small refractive errors of less than 1 D.[3] Recognizing this modest risk factor in addition to the historical risk factors would weigh in the calculation to treat or not.

Well-known are the signs of the pigment dispersion syndrome: the Krukenberg spindle, pigment dusting of the anterior portion of the lens, hyperpigmentation of the trabecular meshwork, and the pathognomonic radial, spokelike transillumination defects in the outer third of the iris. Though less than half of patients with the pigment dispersion syndrome will, with time, go on to pigment dispersion glaucoma,[4] such findings in combination with an elevated pressure and positive family history would likely reinforce any decision to treat high pressures vigorously and to monitor the disc and field status with vigilance.

Though perhaps at the upper end of the age group where malformations of the angle structure would be expected to be manifested as clinical glaucoma, a 45-year-old's eyes could show some anomalous appearance on gonioscopy. Foremost would be a flat peripheral appearance of the iris root (instead of the normal concave configuration), anteriorly inserting at the junction of scleral spur and pigmented meshwork. Sometimes an exuberance of iris processes is seen that spans the spur to insert in the lower meshwork and appears like a carpet wrapped around the entire angle's circumference. Such findings would alert the clinician to the possibility of a "late–juvenile-onset" type of glaucoma with its own clinical peculiarities. For example, this entity frequently does quite poorly with laser trabeculoplasty, yet responds well to trabeculotomy ab externo.

Although not strictly a physical risk factor, the recognition of nerve fiber layer defects by red-free ophthalmoscopy or photography is currently considered a predictor for future glaucomatous defects. The expected normal appearance of a relatively lush nerve fiber layer in this young age group would likely maximize the appreciation of either diffuse or sectoral bundle defects, which may in fact appear in the presence of otherwise normal optic discs and visual fields and presage future damage.

A Uniocular Therapeutic Trial

Assuming that our evaluation has revealed no risk factors other than a one-time reading of 28 mm Hg in both eyes and a history of a brother's glaucoma, it would be prudent to undertake a therapeutic trial with a topical drop in one eye only. This could accomplish three desirable ends. First, it would impress on the patient the potential seriousness of his status as a "glaucoma suspect" and reinforce the admonition to remain under ophthalmologic surveillance at least annually the rest of his life.

Second, a uniocular drop trial would establish the efficacy of that particular agent by using the opposite eye as a reference point. A statistical phenomenon called "regression to the mean" frequently has bearing in measuring IOPs. Quite simply this means there is a certain likelihood that abnormally high pressure readings (such as 28 in this case) will, on a subsequent reading, be lower and closer to the "statistical mean" for IOPs in general. If a topical medicine is truly working, it should cause an obvious difference in pressure between the treated and untreated eye. The magnitude of such a uniocular response would be greater than any possible "crossover" effect from systemic absorption.[5]

Third, a therapeutic trial can help clarify the crucial issue of medical compliance and tolerability. The therapeutic options are relatively restricted in this middle-aged group since miotic therapy is frequently uncomfortable in the presence of a still-accommodating ciliary body. By gently introducing a patient to a regimen in one eye only, topical side effects can often be minimized, the patient can be "bonded" to the ongoing collaborative effort to reduce the risk of glaucoma, and the physician can ascertain whether imperfect compliance with therapy and follow-up requires a more aggressive or definitive approach.

Choice of Trial Medicines

In the absence of any contraindications such as asthma or exercise intolerance, a topical β-blocker would be the first medical choice. Though there is a considerable variability in patient response, a nonspecific β_1- and β_2-blocker such as timolol (Timoptic) or levobunolol (Betagan) could quickly establish whether uniocular β-blockade significantly lowers the pressure. Once this is known, the details of the regimen should be customized: trying once-a-day therapy, a lower concentration, or even a β_1-preferential agent such as betaxolol (Betoptic).

There certainly are a variety of legitimate approaches in selecting a β-blocker, and the one recommended earlier serves the interests of economy of visits—a frequent issue in a large subspecialty referral practice. If a maximal β-blocking agent is insufficient, multiple visits for the refinement of therapy—by either selecting a higher dose, a different schedule, or a different member of the same drug family—can be eliminated. Since the majority of side effects to β-blockade will likely be manifested in the first 6 weeks, the tolerance to this class of agents can be quickly known.

Of similar controversy is the value of adding an epinephrine agent to a β-blocker. A common experience is that though such a drug may sometimes synergize well with a β_1-selective agent such as betaxolol, the combined effect is still of the order obtained with a nonspecific β-blocker alone to which epinephrine is rarely additive in any clinically meaningful sense. In the event that a β-blocker is contraindicated, epinephrine agents are a welcome alternative, though treatment with them is sometimes discontinued because of topical irritation.

More often than not a miotic would be disliked by a 45-year-old patient. There is, however, a wide range of possible responses, depending on the patient's commitment to therapy (and possible fear of not being treated), on his tolerance threshold for predictable side effects, and on any serendipitous advantages with therapy (such as obviating the need for presbyopic correction.) A uniocular trial could begin with pilocarpine 2% drops, beginning nightly with aspirin the first few days and adopting over a few weeks' time to a four-times-a-day regimen. An alternative is to begin with a 4% pilocarpine gel at bedtime (Pilopine), again with clear warnings about local muscular discomfort and miotic interference with customary vision. If initial miotic therapy is acceptable, there are ways to customize a regimen, e.g., using the nightly gel with 3% carbachol in midafternoon for a twice-a-day schedule, trying a sustained-release delivery system (Ocusert) in patients comfortable with contact lenses, etc.

Re-evaluating the Assumptions for Treatment

Should tolerable topical therapy fail to change the pressure profile, there arises the difficult choice of whether to push on to a systemic diuretic (such as low-dose methazolamide [Neptazane] 25 mg twice a day) or laser trabeculoplasty (which would not likely work well in the long run in this young a patient.) Both options put into clear focus the single most difficult problem in any therapeutic trial: when is the pressure "low enough" and how many antiglaucoma agents and maneuvers should be activated for a "glaucoma suspect"?

Quite simply, the decision should *not* depend on the pressures alone. Instead, it should depend on the frequent re-assessment of all currently identified risk factors and physical findings. An appropriate but intensive surveillance scheme for this patient would include computerized full-threshold testing two or three times a year, optic disc and nerve fiber layer evaluation and photography once or twice a year, and pressure measurements every 4 to 6 months. If available, full color testing with the Farnsworth 100-

hue test or contrast sensitivity examination could be obtained as baseline data as well. Should all these tests continually indicate clinical stability of field and nerve function, the antecedent IOPs could well be considered "acceptable," and therapy need not be escalated.

Besides regularly scheduled examination times, there are two other natural stopping points in the therapeutic relationship that allow for re-assessment. One point is when the patient simply cannot tolerate further medications because of local or systemic side effects. At such a juncture, it is appropriate to simply monitor the pressure profile under whatever medicines are acceptable with a clinical surveillance scheme as suggested earlier. Another opportunity to re-evaluate is with a planned 6-week drug "washout" every 12 to 18 months. By discontinuing all therapy, another baseline set of pressures can be identified. Sometimes it seems medicines are having little effect, and treatment with them can be curtailed or stopped. If, on the other hand, there is a marked rise of pressures during the unmedicated observation period, the commitment to therapy is reinforced anew.

Though it is easy indeed to be lulled into substituting "pressure control" for "glaucoma management," the central issue to be perpetually clarified is invariably the same: does a given patient have even the subtlest signs of optic nerve and field damage, or is there only the risk of damage? By constantly asking and reassessing the answers to this question, careful attention and the unfolding of time will reveal whether to proceed either with the qualified treatment of a glaucoma suspect or with the energetic prevention of further ocular disease.

References

1. Armaly MF: Lessons to be learned from the Corroborative Glaucoma Study. *Surv Ophthalmol* 1980; 25:139–144.
2. Anderson DR: Management of elevated intraocular pressure with normal optic discs and visual fields: I. Therapeutic approach based on high risk factors. *Surv Ophthalmol* 1977; 21:479–489.
3. Perkins ES, Phelps CD: Open angle glaucoma, ocular hypertension, low-tension glaucoma and refraction. *Arch Ophthalmol* 1982; 100:1464.
4. Scheie HG, Cameron JD: Pigment dispersion syndrome—A clinical study. *Br J Ophthalmol* 1981; 65:264.
5. Drance SM: The uniocular therapeutic trial in the management of elevated intraocular pressure. *Surv Ophthalmol* 1980; 25:203–205.

Automated Visual Fields—Threshold or Screening?

APPROACH 1

David J. Palmer, M.D.

APPROACH 2

Marshall N. Cyrlin, M.D.

Case 11 _____

Automated Visual Fields— Threshold or Screening?

A 50-year-old woman is found to have intraocular pressures (IOPs) of 30 bilaterally. Her cup-to-disc ratio is 0.8 in each eye. There is an automated perimeter available, but the ophthalmologist must order the type of test.
What program should be selected?

Summary _____

The proliferation of small, easy-to-use, and affordable automated visual field testing equipment has been a great boon to the care of glaucoma patients. Because these tests do not have to be administered by the busy practitioner, a patient is more likely to be tested early in the course of the disease and have the fields followed closely. Unfortunately, the clinician has been forced to learn a new way of ordering and interpreting visual fields. This case presents the question of whether a threshold or screening test is more appropriate in a patient with newly discovered elevated IOP.

Quantitative, full-threshold perimetry is favored by Dr. Palmer. He argues that quantitation of any defects provides greater accuracy and reliability than does a screening test. Having the absolute thresholds at each of the tested locations allows the practitioner to decide which areas are abnormal without relying on the computer to make those decisions based on stored information on "normals."

Dr. Cyrlin points out that the screening test can be used to guide the clinician toward the most appropriate threshold test. While a threshold strategy is necessary for following defects, scotomas can be detected efficiently with a screening test. This has the added benefit of "teaching" the patient how to take the automated test, thus reducing the effect of the learning curve on subsequent threshold tests.

The fatigue factor should not be ignored when choosing a testing strategy. These field examinations are tedious and tiring to the patient, and we must avoid unnecessary testing while maximizing the usefulness of the information that is obtained. Both of the authors make the point that full-threshold testing must be used to *follow* glaucomatous defects.

Approach 1 ————————————

David J. Palmer, M.D.

Glaucoma suspects are those patients with elevated IOP, healthy and symmetrical optic nerves, full visual fields, and the absence of ocular disease secondarily resulting in increased IOP. The risk of glaucomatous evolution in this population ranges from 0% to 9% over 4 to 14 years and is associated with factors such as optic disc abnormalities and size, advancing age, high myopia, a glaucomatous family history, and systemic vascular disease.[1-3] The decision to treat these individuals remains controversial and is justified on the basis of benefits of glaucoma prevention vs. the risk of side effects, cost, inconvenience, and the low rate of glaucoma development.[1-4]

The patient described represents a glaucoma suspect, i.e., the IOP of 30 is greater than normal and the disc cupping, though symmetrical, is large. The patient's age and sex are given, but the refractive state, knowledge of previous IOPs, access to previous disc photographs, or other risk factor information is not presented. Knowledge of the patient's race may also be helpful since blacks are more likely than whites to develop glaucoma[5] and tend to have larger cup-to-disc ratios.[6] According to some authors, physiologically large cups, in general, do not tolerate an increased IOP as well as those with smaller cups.[2, 7]

Visual field changes using manual perimetric methods have occurred in less than 5% of patients with IOPs of 22 to 25 mm Hg who were followed for up to 5 years.[4] This rate of visual field progression increases to 12% to 30% at IOPs of 30 mm Hg.[4, 8] When compared to Goldmann visual field testing, automated techniques can reveal subtle threshold disturbances that may be undetected by tedious and exhaustive manual perimetry. In one series, up to

50% more field defects were noted with automated testing compared with Goldmann perimetry.[9] Of those with automated visual field defects, up to 50% of patients had optic disc damage when examined ophthalmoscopically. Determining whether all changes detected by computerized testing techniques reflect glaucomatous loss is subject to verification by at least two serial testing evaluations.

Most glaucoma visual field automated testing methods concentrate on the central 30 degrees, the location where the majority of changes will occur. In a few instances, peripheral nasal defects may be detected in the absence of central abnormalities.[10] A technique is necessary for obtaining precise measurements of actual thresholds at all test locations to detect the most subtle and early defects as discussed earlier. Quantitative threshold testing is such a technique since the values will provide this essential individualized, reliable, and sensitive information. Additionally, many reports in the literature rely on quantitative threshold approaches for data presentation.

Unlike the screening tests, quantitative threshold testing distinguishes between all defects of varying severity without comparisons to an age-related normal population. The baseline values obtained are actual threshold responses for each point. Assumed levels of normal on a screening examination may underestimate or overestimate the individual's actual threshold since the initial stimulus is usually 4 to 6 dB brighter than an age-related group. Subtle early defects may be missed in fields where the patient's general baseline is higher than *average* normal. Therefore, there is less risk of a quantitative threshold test obscuring the increasing variability of threshold values within (short-term fluctuation) or between (long-term fluctuation) examinations in previously normal areas of the visual field. These signs are considered an early indicator of glaucoma.[11]

The longer test time and potential fatigue of a quantitative threshold field examination compared with the screening examination is balanced by the greater accuracy and reliability of obtained information. Among its advantages, quantitative data collection on all isolated points may be used statistically for determining the reliability of a single visual field (e.g., fluctuation, false positives, false negatives) or for comparative analyses of serial examinations (e.g., long-term fluctuation, linear regression). Threshold depressions due to a cataract or a miotic pupil, for example, can be filtered out mathematically based on the shape of the hill of vision and intratest variability (short-term fluctuation). Statistical probabilities generated from this data indicate the likelihood that the irregularity detected is caused by actual field loss. The data may be plotted graphically to assist in the field analyses. Correlation with clinical parameters is suggested to further substantiate these findings.

Test locations positioned 3 degrees on either side of the meridians facilitate detection of nasal steps above or below the horizontal midline. Positioning test locations on the meridians allows for an accurate assessment of foveal sensitivity and fixation. Merging central and peripheral tests is possible with the automated instruments; however, test time and fatigue become limiting factors. Customized grids can isolate specific sections of the visual field and be used in subsequent analyses. Occasionally, severe visual field loss requires a shift in the fixation point, a larger presenting target, or abandonment of the automated test in favor of manual visual field methods.

Though limited information on the present patient is given, my opinion, based on her IOP and disc cupping, is that she should be treated. Despite a possibly normal visual field in this patient, there is evidence to suggest that a 40% to 50% loss of nerve axons associated with an elevated IOP is necessary before visual field loss is detectable.[12] In addition, a recent prospective series[13] suggests that treatment of glaucoma suspects with a β-blocking agent may result in fewer tension elevations past 30 mm Hg and visual field changes up to 5 years later. Suggested management would be to check tension and visual field values every 3 to 6 months, obtain baseline and yearly disc photos, and further treat for glaucomatous changes as necessary. Until other methods of early glaucoma detection are perfected and available,[14] initiating treatment based on a tension of 30 mm Hg or higher, large cup-to-disc ratios, and preferentially, the quantitative threshold automated visual field is seemingly justifiable.

References

1. Kass MA: When to treat ocular hypertension. *Surv Ophthalmol* 1983; 28(suppl):229–232.
2. Armaly MF, Kolker AE, Levene RZ, et al: Biostatistical analysis of the Collaborative Glaucoma Study. I. Summary report of the risk factors for glaucomatous visual field defects. *Arch Ophthalmol* 1980; 98:2153–2171.
3. Kass MA, Hart WM, Gordon M, et al: Risk factors favoring the development of glaucomatous visual field loss in ocular hypertension. *Surv Ophthalmol* 1980; 25:155–162.
4. Phelps CD: The no treatment approach to ocular hypertension. *Surv Ophthalmol* 1980; 25:175–182.
5. David R, Livingston D, Luntz MH: Ocular hypertension: A comparative follow-up of black and white patients. *Br J Ophthalmol* 1978; 62:676–678.
6. Henry C, Krupin T: Management of ocular hypertension. *Ann Ophthalmol* 1985; 17:518.
7. Shields MB: A revisit: Ocular hypertension, glaucoma suspect, preglaucoma, or glaucoma? *Ann Ophthalmol* 1985; 17:456.
8. Kass MA, Kolker AF, Becker B: Prognostic factors in glaucomatous visual field loss. *Arch Ophthalmol* 1976; 94:1274–1276.
9. Hotchkiss ML, Robin AL, Quigley HA, et al: A comparison of peritest automated perimetry and Goldmann perimetry. *Arch Ophthalmol* 1985; 103:397–403.
10. Caprioli J, Spaeth GL: Static threshold examination of the peripheral nasal visual field in glaucoma. *Arch Ophthalmol* 1985; 103:1150–1154.
11. Whalen WR, Spaeth GL (eds): Basic software: Examination programs and printout results, in *Computerized Visual Fields. What They Are and How to Use Them.* New Jersey, Slack, Inc, 1985, p 65.
12. Quigley HA, Addicks EM, Green WR: Optic nerve damage in human glaucoma: III. Quantitative correlation of nerve fiber loss and visual field defect in glaucoma, ischemic neuropathy, papilledema, and toxic neuropathy. *Arch Ophthalmol* 1982; 100:135–146.
13. Palmer DJ, Remis LL, Hertzmark E, et al: Timolol versus no treatment in the long-term management of glaucoma suspects. *Invest Ophthalmol Vis Sci* 1985; 26:122.
14. Quigley HA: Better methods in glaucoma diagnosis. *Arch Ophthalmol* 1985; 103:186–189.

Approach 2 _____

Marshall N. Cyrlin, M.D.

It has been suggested that a full-threshold test be performed on this patient because it is the most sensitive and specific. This is indeed true if the examiner has knowledge of the patient's visual field from a previously performed manual kinetic or, preferably, automated static perimetric examination. This information would aid the clinician in the selection of a suitable test program based upon the size, location, and depth of any defects present.

The case as presented implies that this patient in particular is one on whom no previous testing has been performed. Under these circumstances there are advantages in not going directly to a full-threshold test as the initial examination. A practical approach would be to perform a full-field or central screening program as a first test.

A screening program is one in which the sensitivity at each test location is compared with a predicted normal value stored in the perimeter or is compared with an estimate made from selected test points during the examination. A single-level screening test would consist of a single suprathreshold stimulus that is used for the entire examination. The results are reported as either seen or unseen points with no information as to the depth of any scotomas that may be present. This is a distinct disadvantage in a patient with an abnormal field since minimal information is derived. A slightly more satisfactory variation would be a threshold-related screening examination in which the single-stimulus intensity is automatically increased as the examination proceeds to more peripheral points. A multiple-level screening examination would be preferable to the single-level test in any patient in whom a field defect is anticipated from the clinical findings.

A multiple-level test further differentiates the abnormal points into areas of relative or absolute scotomas by the presentation of maximal-intensity stimuli to the "missed" points. Examples of this type of test are the Octopus programs 03 or 07 or the Humphrey Field Analyzer Screening programs performed with the "Three-Zone Strategy." Another approach is the Dicon "Two-Zone" program, which performs stepped suprathreshold testing by re-evaluating unseen points at increasing stimulus intensities. Alternatively, screening tests can be performed in which missed points undergo full-threshold analysis as with the "Quantify Defects" option on the Humphrey instrument.

Screening examinations are valuable as an initial examination because they can rapidly identify abnormal fields and provide some information as to the location, size, and relative depth of scotomas. Importantly, they also give the patient an easier first experience with the automated perimeter than would a full-threshold program. Due to the "learning-curve effect," first examinations are generally less reliable than are subsequent ones. For this reason an initial full-threshold examination may not yield a lot more reliable information than would the multiple-level screening test. After an initial assessment has been made, screening tests should not be used for following glaucoma patients. At this point either partial-thresholding or full-thresholding strategies should be employed.

Partial-thresholding programs such as the Octopus program 34 or the Humphrey programs with the "Fast Thresholding" option shorten the test time by performing complete thresholding only on the abnormal points. Partial-thresholding programs should be used with caution, if at all, for long-term follow-up in ocular hypertensive or glaucoma suspect patients. This is due to the possibility that a patient with normal or greater than average thresholds might have a gradual diffuse or localized loss of sensitivity that remains undetected until the thresholds fall below a predetermined level.

An additional option on an initial examination is whether to perform a full-field or just a central screening program. Relative arguments against testing the entire field are the findings that it is not common to find an isolated peripheral defect without a

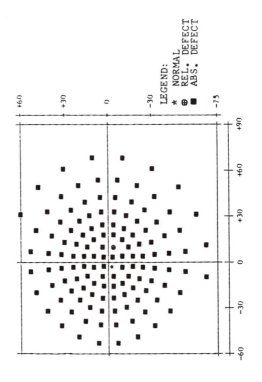

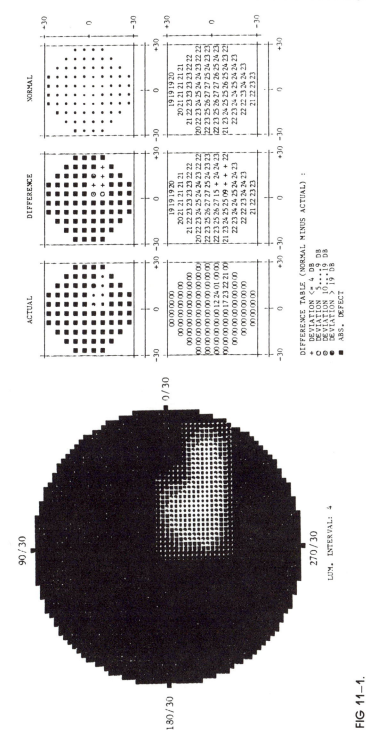

FIG 11–1.
Octopus program 07 multilevel screening test *(top)*. Octopus program 32 central 30-degree thresholding test *(bottom)*.

USER-DEFINED PROGRAM. LABEL: SO4   DATE OF PROGRAM:

USER-DEFINED PROGRAM. LABEL: SO4   DATE OF PROGRAM:

USER-DEFINED PROGRAM:

+10

−10

+10

−10

+10

−10

+10

−10

30

```
        09 14 29
     18 34 30 00 00 24 03
     33 18 35 20 28 27 36
  32 33 33 34 35 36 24 36 36
  33 34 34 35 36 36 36 37 34
```

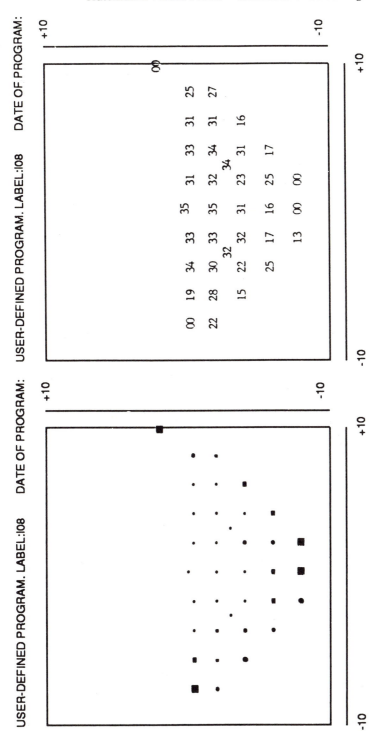

FIG 11–2.
Octopus user-defined custom program of superior 4 degrees and inferior 8 degrees.

central extension and that the accuracy of testing is less in the periphery. The latter point is of greater significance with regard to full-threshold rather than screening programs.

The full-field screening test does serve several important purposes. It can provide information useful for determining the visual function of patients with marked defects in their fields. It can be used to confirm the existence of a questionable defect on the edge of a subsequently performed central-field examination. Of greatest importance is that it allows the clinician to select the most appropriate program for subsequent follow-up with a thresholding program. Most often this will be a central 30-degree test such as the Octopus program 32 or the Humphrey 30-2, which have 6 degrees of resolution. If the screening test indicates that the patient has a 10-degree or smaller central island, then a higher-resolution central examination of the remaining field, such as with the Octopus program 64 or the Humphrey 10-2, should be selected. Finally, if the screening test indicates an irregular or asymmetrical pattern of loss, then a custom-designed test created by a user-defined program may be most appropriate for further follow-up.

The following figures illustrate the previous points. Figure 11–1,A is a screening field of the right eye of a patient with advanced glaucoma. Knowledge of the extent and location of the field loss allows the clinician to avoid performing a worthless routine central 30 degree thresholding test, which is illustrated as an example in Figure 11–1,B. In this time-consuming examination only 7 of 76 test points have measurable sensitivities. Rather than performing an initial routine thresholding test, the more rapid screening test can be used for the selection of custom user-defined examinations of this patient's superior 4 degrees and inferior 8 degrees of remaining field; this is illustrated in Figure 11–2. These high-resolution tests provide much more information and establish a baseline for comparison in the future.

SECTION *IV*

Ocular Inflammation and Trauma

The First Episode of Uveitis—How Extensive a Search?

APPROACH 1

Howard H. Tessler, M.D.

APPROACH 2

Ronald E. Smith, M.D.

Case 12 _____

The First Episode of Uveitis—How Extensive a Search?

A 32-year-old black man complains of redness and pain in both eyes for several days. Examination reveals a moderate anterior-chamber reaction in each eye. There is no previous history of uveitis.

What initial workup is appropriate, and what therapy should be started?

Summary _____

We are often confronted with patients, such as in this case, in whom a "first episode" of iritis or uveitis is present. The questions for the experts concern how extensively to pursue the workup and how best to treat the inflammation.

Dr. Tessler emphasizes the importance of the history in cases of uveitis. The history of the inflammation helps to categorize the problem into acute, recurrent, or chronic iridocyclitis. Bilaterality of the symptoms and the presence of any other systemic complaints also can play a role in helping to define the disease and its prognosis. Laboratory tests are usually not necessary with the first attack.

An extensive laboratory workup also is not recommended by Dr. Smith. However, he points out several special cases in which a limited workup may be helpful. These include cases involving children, instances where ankylosing spondylitis is suspected, and possible instances of sarcoidosis, syphilis, or tuberculosis. In these cases, pinpointing the diagnosis can be helpful in providing prognostic information to the patient and in guiding referral to an appropriate consultant.

Both of the discussants emphasize the importance of fully examining the posterior pole and peripheral part of the retina. Several posterior lesions can cause an anterior-chamber reaction, and in general they are conditions in which early intervention is needed in order to limit the damage. It is well worth waiting an extra few minutes in the office for the pupils to dilate and making a thorough inspection of the fundus prior to initiating therapy.

Approach 1

Howard H. Tessler, M.D.

Initial Evaluation

The most important thing in evaluating this patient, who complains of redness and pain in both eyes, is to get a thorough history. It is important to distinguish acute iritis from chronic iridocyclitis. One must consider the possibility that this patient has had inflammation in both eyes for weeks or months and only recently became symptomatic when he had an acute exacerbation superimposed on a low-grade chronic inflammation. Thus, I would ask whether he has had floaters and spots or vague discomfort in the eyes even predating his recent symptoms.

Acute iritis usually begins abruptly in one eye with severe pain, redness, and photophobia. When inflammation begins bilaterally with only moderate or mild redness, pain, and photophobia, it more likely represents a chronic condition. Thus, although this condition has an acute or short onset, the fact that it is bilateral and that the patient complains of only mild redness and pain implies that this may be the beginning of chronic inflammatory disease.

There are several characteristics that distinguish acute iritis from chronic iritis or iridocyclitis. Acute iritis or iridocyclitis tends to be self-limited in time. The attacks frequently last 2 to 6 weeks. Between episodes of acute iritis the condition of the eye goes into complete remission, and no silent damage occurs. Chronic iritis or iridocyclitis never completely clears. The patient is always at risk for synechia formation and problems with cystoid macular edema (CME).

In the initial evaluation of a patient with a first-time onset of iritis, an extensive laboratory evaluation is probably not warranted because of the expense and because the results frequently do not determine a cause. However, in the initial history taking, it is worth asking the patient about low-back problems. Ankylosing spondylitis is frequently associated with acute iritis. The iritis present with ankylosing spondylitis is usually unilateral; although either eye can be involved, the attacks rarely occur in both eyes simultaneously. In this patient with a bilateral condition, it is unlikely that his disease is related to ankylosing spondylitis. A negative history of arthritis and low-back problems should help rule out this diagnosis. The hallmark symptom of ankylosing spondylitis is stiffness after inactivity. These patients frequently have pain on arising in the morning. They have difficulty sleeping late in the morning and have to get out of bed and move about to relieve stiffness. If they sit in a chair too long, their back stiffens, and they have difficulty unbending.

HLA-B27, part of the major histocompatibility complex, is a useful marker for a genetic tendency to both acute iritis and ankylosing spondylitis. There is an inherited tendency to develop iritis and ankylosing spondylitis. It is worth asking the patient not only whether other family members have had iritis but also whether there are back problems in the family. Male family members especially may have low-back problems. Ankylosing spondylitis tends to be more severe in men than in women. However, in this patient one would not highly suspect HLA-B27 and ankylosing spondylitis since HLA-B27 is not a common antigen in blacks.

Sarcoidosis, on the other hand, is a common cause of iritis and iridocyclitis in black patients. Ocular sarcoidosis frequently presents subacutely and bilaterally. It is valuable to ask the patient whether he has ever been diagnosed as having sarcoidosis. He should be asked about symptoms or lesions affecting the skin or the lungs and told that while sarcoidosis can involve any part of the body it most commonly tends to affect the skin, lungs, and eyes.

Further questioning might elicit a history of oral or genital ulcers, venereal disease, and urinary tract problems. This information might implicate rare diseases such as Behçet's syndrome, syphilis, or Reiter's syndrome.

If the patient gives positive answers to these history questions, one should suspect that he might have an underlying systemic disease that could be associated with his eye problem. If the answers are negative, one could assume, until more extensive laboratory evaluations are done, that he has idiopathic inflammation.

Fuchs' heterochromic iridocyclitis (FHI) is a remote possibility. FHI usually is unilateral and asymptomatic as far as redness and pain are concerned. However, bilateral FHI is sometimes reported and thus probably worth considering as a diagnosis in this patient.

Examination is very important. I always stress the importance of a best-corrected visual acuity. Frequently CME occurs with iritis, especially chronic iritis. Media opacities such as cells and flare rarely, on their own, cause much diminishment of vision. Thus, if the visual acuity is less than 20/20, one should at least consider the possibility that CME may be present.

It is important to turn on the room lights and stand back and look at the patient's eyes and face. As I mentioned earlier, FHI is a diagnostic possibility. Heterochromia can be more easily discovered by looking at both eyes simultaneously. In a dark brown–eyed patient heterochromia can be quite subtle. Scleritis also might be missed if the patient is too readily placed at the slit lamp and the whole eye not evaluated.

Slit-lamp examination is most important. If keratic precipitates (KPs) are present, their size and distribution should be noted. In FHI the KPs are fine and stellate and diffusely cover the entire cornea. Large granulomatous KPs occur with sarcoidosis, and fine nongranulomatous KPs occur in HLA-B27 disease.

Because this patient may require a return visit, it is important to grade the cells and flare rather than recording "moderate" anterior-chamber reaction. Grading the reaction (1 +, 2 +, etc.) makes comparison from visit to visit more accurate.

The presence of synechiae is important. A lack of synechiae might be a sign of an entity such as FHI. The presence of iris nodules might indicate a granulomatous etiology.

The anterior portion of the vitreous will help determine

whether the patient has an iritis or iridocyclitis. If the cellular densities are equal or greater in the anterior part of the vitreous than those in the anterior chamber, one must assume a cyclitis is present. If most of the inflammation is in the anterior chamber and very little is in the anterior portion of the vitreous, one might call this a pure iritis.

The intraocular pressure must be checked. Often in acute and chronic iritis the intraocular pressure is low due to ciliary body infiltration and decreased secretion of aqueous. However, there are times when there is so much debris clogging the trabecular meshwork that the pressure is elevated. Also, because this patient most likely will be placed on a regimen of topical corticosteroids, he must be monitored for the possibility of a glaucoma response.

Every new patient with iritis needs a fundus examination with pupillary dilation. Although I am assuming this patient has a pure iritis or iridocyclitis, it is very important not to miss a lesion in the fundus that could cause an anterior segment reaction. A toxoplasmic granuloma in the retina could, via anterior segment spillover, be the source of an iritis. Both direct and indirect ophthalmoscopy should be performed. Peripheral granulomas could be missed without doing this complete examination. Also, the pars plana should be evaluated for the possibility of pars planitis. Last, in this day of acquired immunodeficiency syndrome (AIDS), the patient might have an opportunistic viral retinitis that could present as an iritis. Even in the absence of AIDS, the acute retinal necrosis syndrome may present initially as an iritis.

Because I suspect sarcoidosis in this particular patient, evidence of periphlebitis such as focal or linear sheathing of the retinal veins is important. Tiny focal granulomas in the choroid or retina may also be significant. Snowball opacities over the peripheral inferior part of the retina are suggestive of sarcoid.

After completing the evaluation, I would tell the patient that he has acute iritis, which is usually of short duration, but that I am somewhat concerned he may have a chronic inflammatory condition in his eye that might persist for months or even years. Unless there were a focal granuloma or a specific finding in the fundus to account for his eye disease, I would express uncertainty at this stage as to how long the disease will be active. His visual prognosis is also uncertain, but at present his eye problem is mild, and he probably will maintain good vision. However, it is important, without alarming the patient, to tell him that he has more than simple "pink eye." He should understand that he has a disease that is affecting the inside of the eye and potentially might be visually threatening. I inform such patients that it is important to follow instructions and to return for further evaluation.

I often use arthritis as an analogy. I tell patients that, although the treatment may not cure the disease, we try to prevent deformities in the eye much as one tries to prevent deformities in the joints when people are treated for arthritis.

Treatment

For the moderate anterior chamber reaction that is described in this patient, I would initially prescribe topical corticosteroids. I recommend 1% prednisolone acetate suspension four times a day. This suspension seems to give good penetration and is probably somewhat more effective than the solutions. I would first explain the side effects of topical corticosteroids (e.g., cataracts, glaucoma, and susceptibility to secondary infection by viruses or other germs). I would reassure him that, as long as he keeps his appointments, close follow-up will minimize side effects, especially in the short term.

If there are synechiae or ciliary spasm, I usually prescribe cycloplegic therapy for the patient. For the moderate amount of inflammation described in this patient, 5% homatropine once or twice a day is probably adequate. However, if the patient has severe, painful, ciliary spasm, a short course of atropine might be indicated. If there is evidence of synechia formation, an attempt in the office to break the synechiae with frequent dilation would be in order. However, this case is described as moderate, and I would not anticipate a tremendous amount of synechiae. If there is an abnormally high intraocular pressure, a topical β-blocker could also be used.

If the patient had good visual acuity (20/40 or better) in addition to only moderate anterior-chamber reaction, he probably would be seen again in 1 week. In the case of severe inflammation with fibrin or synechia formation or diminished visual acuity, the patient should be seen sooner (1 or 2 days). If in 1 week the patient has improved, the dosage of drops can be gradually tapered and then stopped. In standard acute iritis the inflammation is self-limited at 2 to 6 weeks, and the disease should go into complete remission. If, as I suspect, this bilateral-onset disease is the beginning of a chronic inflammatory condition, the patient may need eyedrops for many months or even years.

In patients with chronic iridocyclitis permanent breakdown of the blood-aqueous barrier usually occurs. The anterior chambers in these chronic cases may never completely clear. Thus, I am usually reasonably happy to keep the anterior chamber reaction at 1 + or 2 + cell and flare as long as the patient is comfortable and visual acuity remains good. I would not overtreat someone who has chronic ocular inflammation.

After several weeks or months, if this patient's uveitis is not going into remission or he develops chronic CME or does not do well, it is probably appropriate to do a more thorough laboratory evaluation.

Bibliography

1. Godfrey WA: Acute anterior uveitis in Tessler HH, Duane TO, Jaeger EA (eds): *Clinical Ophthalmology*, vol 4. Philadelphia, Harper & Row, Publishers, Inc, 1987, pp 1–11.
2. Godfrey WA: Chronic iridocyclitis, in Tessler HH, Duane TO, Jaeger EA (eds): *Clinical Ophthalmology*, vol 4. Philadelphia, Harper & Row, Publishers, Inc, 1987, pp 1–13.
3. Smith RE, Nozik RA: *Uveitis: A Clinical Approach to Diagnosis and Management*. Baltimore, Williams & Wilkins, 1983, pp 2–72.
4. Tessler HH: Uveitis, in Peyman GA, Sanders DR, Goldberg MF (eds): *Principles and Practice of Ophthalmology*, Philadelphia, WB Saunders Co, 1980, pp 1554–1590.

Approach 2 _____

Ronald E. Smith, M.D.

In general, my approach to the first episode of "uveitis" depends on the location of the inflammation. The workup of a patient with a retinitis or diffuse uveitis (e.g., pars planitis) would be different from that of a patient with primary iridocyclitis. Since the case under discussion is an iridocyclitis, the following discussion relates specifically to the workup and management of the first episode of iridocyclitis.

If the first episode of iridocyclitis is unilateral and does not include large mutton-fat KPs ("granulomatous"), I generally do not embark on a systemic evaluation. While I certainly vigorously treat the first episode of iridocyclitis as outlined later, I reserve any "workup" for patients with recurrent episodes of iridocyclitis or patients with bilateral, active iridocyclitis, as represented by the current case.

The Workup

The evaluation of iridocyclitis depends to some extent on the age of the patient. For example, in a child with a chronic or acute iridocyclitis, one of the most common associations is juvenile rheumatoid arthritis (JRA) or one of its variants. In such cases, an antinuclear antibody test and a knee x-ray are important (the knee is the most commonly involved joint in JRA). More importantly, referral to a pediatrician or pediatric rheumatologist for a thorough evaluation is preferred. In children with iridocyclitis, it is also important to rule out unusual causes such as sarcoid, syphilis, and tuberculosis (see a later discussion).

In all cases of iridocyclitis—adult or childhood—it is most important to thoroughly examine the fundus of the eye with a dilated pupil in order to rule out the possibility of a retinitis or retinal vasculitis. It is not uncommon for such posterior conditions to cause significant anterior chamber reaction and even hypopyon, which leads to the presumptive diagnosis of a primary iridocyclitis when, in fact, the iridocyclitis is actually *secondary* to the underlying retinitis. This is especially typical of active toxoplasmic retinochoroiditis. A thorough ocular examination including indirect ophthalmoscopy is therefore essential in the workup of any patient with iridocyclitis.

In adults with iridocyclitis, the workup again focuses on systemic syndromes that may be associated with rheumatologic conditions. One of the most common causes of recurrent and acute iridocyclitis in young males (as exemplified by the case under consideration) is ankylosing spondylitis. Usually, the iridocyclitis is not active in both eyes simultaneously, but I have seen such cases. Obtain a sacroiliac x-ray in such cases since patients may have early ankylosing spondylitis in the absence of any significant symptoms or objective findings of this potentially disabling form of arthritis. Early referral to a rheumatologist for diagnosis and therapy may help reduce the systemic morbidity of this condition.

HLA-B27 testing may be helpful in categorizing iridocyclitis but is not useful from the therapeutic standpoint. In most cases of iridocyclitis, I do obtain this test in order to diagnose and establish a prognosis. HLA-B27 antigen is present in most cases of iridocyclitis associated with ankylosing spondylitis or Reiter's disease. There is also a form of iridocyclitis in which the only abnormality appears to be the presence of the HLA-B27 antigen. This has a variable prognosis but may be important from the diagnostic standpoint.

It is equally important to rule out sarcoidosis in individuals with acute and chronic iridocyclitis in both eyes, especially in black patients in whom this particular disease is more prevalent. Appropriate testing would include a determination of the levels of angiotensin-converting enzyme and serum lysozyme, chest x-ray, and possibly a limited gallium scan. A combination of angiotensin-converting enzyme assay, chest x-ray, and a limited gallium scan will detect the majority of cases of sarcoidosis associated with iridocyclitis. Additional clinical features that may point to the diagnosis of sarcoid include the presence of large mutton fat KPs, iris nodules, conjuctival granulomas, and retinal periphlebitis.

With the resurgence of venereal disease in this country, it is always important to rule out the possibility of syphilitic iridocyclitis in patients with a severe bilateral first episode of iridocyclitis. One of the most useful tests in such cases is the MHA-TP or fluorescent treponemal antibody absorption test (FTA-ABS). The VDRL response may be negative in such patients; therefore, I generally do not obtain this test but prefer the former studies. I refer these patients to the appropriate internist, dermatologist, or neurologist for consideration of cerebral spinal fluid studies prior to systemic therapy.

In addition to syphilis, it is important to rule out tuberculosis. While rare, I have seen a few cases over the past 10 years. These eyes can be salvaged if the disease is recognized and treated early. Tuberculin skin testing and chest x-ray are appropriate studies.

Management of Iridocyclitis

I manage the first episode of acute iridocyclitis much as I manage every subsequent episode of recurrent and acute iridocyclitis. The mainstay of therapy is topical corticosteroids. Most cases will respond quite well to hourly doses of any form of full-strength topical corticosteroid drops; I generally use dexamethasone phosphate, but have used other preparations as well. I try to vigorously dilate the pupil during the first office visit to be certain that any synechiae are broken. It is rare to have to resort to subconjunctival dilating agents for this purpose. I prefer the use of short-acting or medium-acting dilators and cycloplegics in cases of acute iridocyclitis rather than long-acting cycloplegics such as atropine or scopolamine. With use of the long-acting agents, the pupil may become "stuck" in the dilated position rather than in the miotic position. I usually use cyclopentolate 1% or tropicamide 0.5% drops three or four times a day, or more often if necessary, in the early treatment of acute iridocyclitis.

I see patients again within 5 to 7 days after the initiation of therapy and begin to taper the topical corticosteroid and the topical cycloplegic dosage according to the response of the anterior-chamber reaction. If the inflammation is extremely severe and poorly responsive to topical medication after 5 to 7 days, I then use subconjunctival or sub-Tenon long-acting corticosteroid therapy; I do not use short-acting corticosteroids for periocular injection. In the most severe cases, I have used pulsed high-dose systemic prednisone in a range of 60 to 100 mg/day for a week in the average adult patient.

Summary

As discussed at the outset, the first episode of unilateral acute iridocyclitis without large mutton-fat KPs is managed with high-dose topical steroids and cycloplegics, and I do not pursue any type of systemic evaluation. Corticosteroid drops are generally effective in most cases. However, in bilateral iridocyclitis or chronic iridocyclitis, I suggest the systemic evaluation outlined earlier. It is most important to rule out the possibility of a retinitis or retinal vasculitis during the initial evaluation in such cases so as to be certain that you are not dealing with a "spillover" iridocyclitis from a posterior segment form of inflammation.

Bibliography

1. Smith RE, Nozik R: *Uveitis: A Clinical Approach to Diagnosis and Management.* Baltimore, Williams & Wilkins, 1983, pp 72–75.

Chronic Sarcoid Uveitis—Surgical or Medical Management?

APPROACH 1

Henry J. Kaplan, M.D.

APPROACH 2

Robert B. Nussenblatt, M.D.

Case 13 —————————————

Chronic Sarcoid Uveitis—Surgical or Medical Management?

A 38-year-old man has had chronic sarcoid uveitis for 3 years. He has been treated with topical and periocular steroids. Currently, his treatment regimen consists of topical steroid drops six times per day and prednisone, 20 mg every morning. Attempts to taper his prednisone dose under this level have failed because of worsening of cystoid macular edema (CME).

What treatment options are available at this point?

Summary

Patients with chronic uveitis are among the most difficult and frustrating in our practices. Frequently the inflammation appears to have been quieted, only to have it return with a vengeance when tapering of medications is begun. In this case of sarcoidosis, two experts discuss their approaches: either surgical or medical management.

Dr. Kaplan begins his discussion with a review of the systemic and ocular manifestations of sarcoidosis. He then describes his therapeutic approach, culminating in the indications for pars plana vitrectomy for recalcitrant cases. There is now experimental evidence that provides some explanations for why this long-advocated approach may be helpful.

The importance of a detailed search for the cause of reduced vision in this patient is emphasized by Dr. Nussenblatt. One should not assume that CME is the only cause of the visual deficit. Dr. Nussenblatt details his medical approach and points out that there is evidence that, once CME is established, vitrectomy is not a useful approach.

Both of the discussants stress that the use of corticosteroids should be continued if they are working and continue to be tolerated. Of all the available immunosuppressive agents available, prednisone is probably the safest and certainly is the drug with which we have the most experience.

Approach 1 _____

Henry J. Kaplan, M.D.

The history is that of a 38-year-old man with chronic sarcoid uveitis for 3 years who has been receiving a maintenance regimen of prednisone (20 mg each morning) because of recurrent CME. The question posed is what treatment options are available at this point? Since sarcoidosis is a systemic disease with protean manifestations, the discussion will first begin with a brief overview of this multisystem disorder.

Diagnosis of Sarcoidosis

Although ocular sarcoidosis is generally thought to be part of a multisystem granulomatous disorder, it is frequently difficult to demonstrate characteristic lesions elsewhere in the body. Nevertheless, it is important to try to establish the correct diagnosis. Since the etiology of systemic sarcoidosis is unknown, the patient will be relegated to treatment with nonspecific inflammatory medications rather than specific curative chemotherapy, which could be harmful in infectious uveitis.

Systemic sarcoidosis presents in one of three forms:

1. As asymptomatic pulmonary disease detected on a routine chest x-ray and requiring no therapy in 40%.
2. As acute benign disease with erythema nodosum and pulmonary hilar lymphadenopathy but no constitutional symptoms.
3. As chronic severe disease, the least common form, associated with progressive pulmonary parenchymal damage and extrapulmonary manifestations.

The acute, benign form of systemic sarcoidosis spontaneously resolves in 2 years, and the most troublesome aspect may be acute anterior uveitis. Since these patients have no constitutional symptoms or permanent sequelae, they are not treated with systemic medications. In contrast, patients with the chronic severe form frequently require systemic treatment.

Multiple organ systems may be involved in systemic sarcoidosis—up to 50% of patients have respiratory symptoms, with mediastinal or pulmonary hilar adenopathy found on chest x-ray in 90%; erythema nodosum, typically on the front of the legs, may occur in up to two thirds of female patients; 5% present with osteoporosis, cystic rarefaction, and cortical thinning of the phalanges, metacarpals, and metatarsals; an acute transient severe polyarthritis has been reported in 38%; about 5% experience central nervous system involvement, usually the result of a basal granulomatous meningitis; and extrathoracic lymphadenopathy, particularly of the cervical lymph nodes, occurs in 75% and splenomegaly in 50%.

Multiple diagnostic tests are helpful in confirming the presence of systemic sarcoidosis:

1. Chest x-ray, which may reveal hilar or paratracheal lymphadenopathy and/or pulmonary infiltration.
2. Biopsy of involved tissue.
    a. Transbronchial or open-lung biopsy both have a high positive yield. Bronchoalveolar lavage is a relatively new diagnostic tool that has also been used to assess the activity of inflammatory disease.
    b. Scalene or supraclavicular lymph node.
    c. Skin nodule (e.g., the eyelid), conjunctival nodule, or the palpebral portion of the lacrimal gland. Blind biopsy of the conjunctiva has not yielded worthwhile information.
3. Determination of the levels of serum calcium (10%), angiotensin-converting enzyme (75%) and/or lysozyme, although elevated serum levels are not pathognomonic for sarcoidosis.
4. Gallium 67 scan of the lung and lacrimal gland. The radioisotope is taken up by sarcoid macrophages but not by normal ones.

A diagnosis of ocular sarcoidosis should not be made without the characteristic clinical and laboratory findings of systemic sarcoidosis.

Ocular Disease In Sarcoidosis

Ocular involvement in sarcoidosis occurs in up to 50% of cases. Although rarely of practical importance, keratoconjunctivitis sicca is observed in 19%, usually in association with an enlarged lacrimal gland. However, the most common form of ocular involvement is uveitis, in particular, panuveitis.

Three different patterns of intraocular inflammation are encountered.

1. Acute anterior uveitis, usually observed in acute benign systemic disease, is indistinguishable from acute anterior uveitis of other causes, has a very good prognosis, and responds promptly to topical prednisolone, 1% (or the equivalent), and mydriasis.

2. Chronic granulomatous uveitis, frequently seen in chronic severe systemic disease, is associated with mutton-fat keratic precipitates, synechiae formation, and secondary glaucoma occur. Vascularized nodules of the iris stroma may be seen, particularly in the anterior chamber angle, which predispose to peripheral anterior synechiae. At the pupillary margin Koeppe nodules may form. The posterior segment of the eye often also shows signs of inflammation, i.e., panuveitis.

3. Posterior segment inflammation can occur and can have many manifestations—snowball vitreous opacities, which upon settling to the inferior pars plana may mimic the "snowbank" of intermediate uveitis (pars planitis); papilledema and optic nerve granuloma formation (7%); periphlebitis, with the classic but rare candle-wax drippings; preretinal and/or subretinal neovascularization; and choroidal granuloma formation.

Although a combination of ocular findings will suggest sarcoidosis, it is certainly not specific. In a patient without other evidence of sarcoid the diagnosis can only be suspected, not conclusively established.

Treatment of Ocular Sarcoid

The use of corticosteroids is beneficial in ocular sarcoid and usually does not require other medical and/or surgical intervention. This is particularly true of acute anterior uveitis and even chronic granulomatous uveitis when there is no posterior segment inflammation. Topical prednisolone acetate, 1%, and mydriasis with a short-acting, mydriatic-cycloplegic medication (e.g., cyclopentolate HCl [Cyclogyl], 1%) to maintain movement of the pupil and prevent posterior synechiae formation is all that is required.

However, posterior segment inflammation will often result in the development of both a posterior subcapsular cataract (PSC) and CME, either of which may decrease vision. Periocular (subtenon) corticosteroids (triamcinolone acetonide [Kenalog] 40 mg/cc) may be helpful in the management of these complications, but since the disease is frequently chronic as well as bilateral, oral corticosteroids (prednisone) are needed. The two most common indications for prednisone therapy are the development and/or progression of a PSC cataract and decreased vision (to 20/30 or less) secondary to CME.

Prednisone therapy should be initiated with either 80 or 120 mg/day in four divided doses. Therapy should be continued until a maximal therapeutic response is obtained for at least 2 weeks. The dosage of prednisone can then be slowly tapered—first to alternate-day therapy in a single consolidated dose (e.g., 80 or 120 mg), with subsequent weekly lowering of the total dose until the minimal effective dose is determined. If 20 mg of prednisone every morning is required to prevent worsening of CME and preservation of vision, the patient should be maintained on this regimen, with periodic attempts (every 6 months) at lowering the dosage further.

The only therapeutic options available are either immunosuppressive medical therapy or pars plana vitrectomy surgery. Immunosuppression, with either first-generation cytotoxic drugs such as azathioprine or second-generation immunosuppressive drugs such as cyclosporine, is rarely indicated in sarcoidosis. The disease most often responds to prednisone therapy, and the toxic effects of these drugs are very serious. Furthermore, sarcoidosis is already characterized by an abnormality in T-cell function, i.e., decreased delayed-type hypersensitivity to common skin test antigens (tuberculin, mumps, *Candida*, etc.), so further systemic immunosuppression may present unwarranted risks.

The beneficial effects of pars plana vitrectomy in uveitis were first demonstrated by Dr. J. Diamond and myself in 1978 in patients with chronic uveitis of various etiologies with secondary cataract. Our experience established several important principles:

1. Eyes with chronic uveitis can tolerate pars plana vitrectomy and/or lensectomy quite well.
2. Re-establishment of a clear visual axis in these eyes results in a marked improvement in visual acuity.
3. Following surgery the course of uveitis was frequently altered so that recurrent episodes of uveitis were both less frequent and less severe.

Additional experience has since been gained by many vitreoretinal surgeons that has confirmed these observations. The indications for vitrectomy surgery in posterior inflammation in ocular sarcoidosis are as follows:

1. Opacification of the visual axis from vitreous debris sufficient to account for the decreased vision.
2. Intolerance to the side effects of systemic corticosteroid therapy.
3. Unresponsiveness to systemic corticosteroid therapy, which can be manifested as either progression of a PSC cataract or persistence of CME.

It is important to distinguish between the progression of a PSC cataract as a side effect of prednisone therapy rather than persistent posterior inflammation. Likewise, it is imperative to intervene relatively early in the course of visually disabling CME before there are irreversible alterations in the macula.

I have recently operated upon four eyes with ocular sarcoidosis and a PSC cataract in which a combined extracapsular cataract extraction, insertion of a posterior chamber intraocular lens, and pars plana vitrectomy were performed. All four eyes tolerated the surgical procedure very well, with resultant vision of 20/30 or better. It is important to accurately assess the cause of decreased vision in such patients because long-standing irreversible CME will not be improved by vitrectomy surgery. Following the operation, the course of uveitis in each of these patients was improved.

Why should vitrectomy surgery alter the course of posterior uveitis in sarcoidosis or other types of uveitis? Although the beneficial effect of vitrectomy surgery in chronic uveitis was observed in 1978, it was not until recently that the probable explanation became apparent. Streilein and colleagues have just demonstrated the presence of a soluble factor in the aqueous humor that can suppress the immune response to antigen-specific or antigen-nonspecific lymphocyte proliferation. We have extended these observations to demonstrate the absence of such a factor in normal vitreous, with its appearance in the vitreous cavity following vitrectomy surgery. Thus, it is very possible that the diminished inflammation in chronic uveitis following vitreous surgery is the result of the permeation of this soluble suppressor factor throughout the vitreous cavity.

The postoperative care of such patients is relatively simple. High-dose prednisone therapy, which is started just prior to surgery, is slowly tapered to the minimally effective dose. Frequently it can be totally discontinued. Topical corticosteroid and antibiotic medications are managed as in routine vitreous surgery.

Bibliography

1. Diamond JG, Kaplan HJ: Lensectomy and vitrectomy for complicated cataract secondary to uveitis. *Arch Ophthalmol* 1978; 96:1798–1804.
2. Dinning WJ: *Systemic Inflammatory Disease and the Eye.* Bristol, Wright, 1987, pp 39–58.
3. Kaiser CJ, Ksander B, Streilein JW: Inhibition of lymphocyte proliferative responses to alloantigens by aqueous humor. *Invest Ophthalmol Vis Sci* 1987; 28(suppl):41.

Approach 2 _____

Robert B. Nussenblatt, M.D.

The history is that of an adult male who has had sarcoid uveitis for 3 years and "chronic" CME that worsens with attempts at tapering the dosage of his daily prednisone. The continued administration of immunosuppressive therapy should be based on several factors, including the degree of ocular inflammatory activity, the reasonable hope for "reversibility" of the lesion with continued immunosuppressive therapy, as well as the secondary problems besides CME that can affect the vision in patients with sarcoid uveitis.

Evaluation of the Sarcoid Uveitis Patient

In patients with chronic inflammatory disease, the treating physician runs the risk of concentrating on a single aspect of the inflammatory disease, usually the presence of cell and flare. It is important to evaluate the ocular condition on a regular basis in order to determine whether continued therapy is useful: should it be stopped or altered? Several items need to be considered:

1. It is imperative that the visual acuity be tested in a standard fashion each time the patient comes for a visit. So much of the decision making is dependent on this measurement, and frequently it is performed with the least amount of attention.

2. The amount of intraocular inflammatory activity needs to be assessed. Is there evidence of an active inflammatory disease posteriorly? We have used vitreal haze, which we can then compare to a series of standardized photos[1] as our indicators of vitreal

activity. Though we note the number of cells in the vitreous, the haze for us is the indicator of activity. If there is no vitreal haze or cells, then one must be suspicious as to the reversibility of the decreased vision and as to whether the cause is due to an inflammatorily driven process.

3. A detailed evaluation of the retina is periodically called for. Of particular import would be the presence of a choroidal granuloma, which can appear anywhere and could be the source of the disease in vision. Further, the cystoid edema should be evaluated. Generally, we find the Hruby lens quite good for this evaluation, particularly if fluorescein angiography is to be performed the same day. It is important to rule out the presence of a macular hole. Additionally, a careful evaluation of the posterior pole for evidence of hemorrhage is very important since chronic inflammatory disease can lead to subretinal neovascularization. Additionally, preretinal membranes are often seen.

4. Laser interferometry is a simple test that is very helpful in assessing whether aggressive immunotherapy will be helpful in restoring vision.[2] If the visual acuity as taken on the standard Snellen or Early Treatment of Diabetic Retinopathy Study (ETDRS) chart is 20/40 or less, we would ideally like to see an improvement in laser-predicted acuity of at least three lines. We have found that 86% of patients in whom the laser interferometer predicted an improvement of three or more lines did improve.

5. Any question of optic nerve disease needs to be ruled out as well. Though certainly not indicated for all cases, it is sometimes necessary to consider the following tests: computed axial tomographic (CAT) scan of the orbit, visually evoked response, or tomography of the orbit.

6. The degree of lenticular opacity is of great import as well. We have noted a rather dramatic worsening of cataract in these patients over a short period of time. Here as well, a laser acuity determination can be most helpful in assessing the situation.

7. A fluorescein angiogram will be helpful in assessing whether continued therapy is indicated. It is clear that angiography is mandatory if subretinal neovascularization is present, but it will also help in the evaluation of cystoid edema. The presence of late staining on the angiogram in a typical "petaloid" appearance of

CME does not necessarily indicate for us that the vision is decreased because of this. We would look at the early frames of the angiogram when the edge of the capillary-free zone is best defined. Using a stereoscopic reading device (a "map reader" is ideal) we measure the amount of retinal thickness in the macula. It is this sequela of CME that appears to be associated with a decrease in vision.[3] It should be mentioned that some patients will have no vitreal activity but evidence of macular cysts on clinical examination. These lesions may not fill with fluorescein. This would indicate that the CME is structurally fixed and no longer driven by the inflammatory response. Therefore, further immunosuppression would not be indicated.

Treatment

After the preceding evaluation, we will assume that the CME is the cause for the drop in visual acuity. In deciding which therapeutic approach to use, one also needs to know whether this is a bilateral or unilateral condition and by how much the vision falls when the 20 mg of prednisone is decreased. Assuming that the patient has no untoward effects of the steroid, I would consider leaving him at 20 mg/day for an extended period of time (2 to 3 months).

If the vision is good (>20/40) and the vision falls 1 to 2 lines, I probably would not be alarmed. If I initiated a taper of the prednisone dosage, I would do it very slowly. If the patient's vision has demonstrated profound sensitivity to prednisone dosage reduction previously, I would decrease the dosage by $2^1/_2$ mg and not change the dosage for 2 to 3 months. Therefore, the tapering period could take up to 1 year.

The patient in question is using topical steroids as well. If this is for anterior segment inflammation, I would continue, but if it is for the treatment of the CME, I would stop administration since the effect of steroid on the posterior pole in phakic individuals via this route would be minimal.

This patient, whose disease is controlled with 20 mg of prednisone per day, probably does not need a change in his therapeutic regimen. However, if he needed to stop taking systemic prednisone rapidly, then a series of periocular injections of 1/2 cc Depo-Medrol, 3 to 4 of them separated by 10 to 14 days, might be considered. If this approach improved the visual acuity, then repeat injections every 5 to 6 months could be tried. If the patient required an injection a month, I would not continue this mode of therapy for any extended period of time.

If after a short taper there is a dramatic increase in inflammatory activity in both eyes with a dramatic drop in vision, then other approaches might be considered:

1. Returning to a dosage of 1 to $1^1/_2$ mg/kg of prednisone with a repeat slow taper is one approach.

2. Beginning cyclosporine at 4 to 5 mg/kg combined with a dosage of prednisone from 10 to 15 mg/day should be considered only after a general medical evaluation with special emphasis on the presence of renal disease or hypertension.

3. Another approach has been the use of high-dose pulse steroids ($^1/_2$ to 1 gm given intravenously over 12 to 24 hours). Without the addition of a moderate dosage of systemic steroids, the effect between "boluses" does not appear to last. Therefore, I do not see much advantage to this approach.

4. The use of cytotoxic agents has been used in the United States only for a very limited number of sarcoid uveitis patients. The potential for serious side effects would make me very reticent to use this approach.

5. The use of vitrectomy as an immunosuppressive approach has been raised. Limon and colleagues have reported that in over 100 uveitis cases, once the CME was established, vitrectomy was not useful as a therapeutic approach.[4] This has been our experience as well.

References

1. Nussenblatt RB, Palestine AG, Chan CC, et al: Standardization of vitreal inflammatory activity in intermediate and posterior uveitis. *Ophthalmology* 1985; 92:467–471.
2. Palestine AG, Alter GJ, Chan CC, et al: Laser interferometry and vis-

ual prognosis in uveitis. *Ophthalmology* 1985; 92:1567–1569.

3. Nussenblatt RB, Kaufman SC, Palestine AG, et al: Macular thickening and visual acuity: Measurement in patients with cystoid macular edema. *Ophthalmology*, 1987; 94:1134–1139.

4. Limon S, Bloch-Michel E, Furia M: 100 vitrectomies in uveitis, in Saari KM (ed): *Uveitis Update*. Amsterdam, Excerpta Medica, 1984, pp 521–524.

Traumatic Hyphema—
Home or Away?

APPROACH 1

Thomas A. Deutsch, M.D.

APPROACH 2

Paul E. Romano, M.D.

Case 14 _____

Traumatic Hyphema—Home or Away?

A 7-year-old child is brought to the emergency room after being hit in the left eye with a jump rope. His right eye is normal, but the left eye has a 2-mm hyphema with a visual acuity of 20/70. No other abnormalities are found.

The parents would like to take the child home and promise bed rest and frequent follow-up with the ophthalmologist. Is this the proper treatment?

Summary _____

The patient described in this case suffered a potentially tragic accident. The question being raised is whether the tragedy will be compounded if the child is not admitted to the hospital.

In my discussion of the case, I emphasize the importance of the complications of hyphema as a guide to therapy. With regard to hospitalization, the important point is that our understanding of the natural course of traumatic hyphema as well as response to treatment is derived from inpatients. Until the same rigorous studies are performed on outpatients, I will continue advocating hospitalization for all hyphema patients and insisting on it when the patient is a child.

Dr. Romano eloquently argues the case for the use of systemic medications to prevent secondary hemorrhage. While systemic treatment still does not seem to have become commonplace in the general ophthalmic community, readers should be aware that the majority of researchers in the field of ocular trauma advocate the use of either systemic corticosteroids or an antifibrinolytic agent.

Both of the discussions of this case make the point that the initial size of the hyphema is not of value in predicting whether a secondary hemorrhage will occur. In other words, the ophthalmologist cannot use the size of a child's hyphema to decide whether an aggressive or casual approach to treatment should be employed, and therefore all children should be hospitalized.

Approach 1

Thomas A. Deutsch, M.D.

The history is that of a child with a traumatic hyphema. Because the management of these cases is aimed at the prevention and treatment of complications, this discussion will begin with a description of those complications.

Early Complications

The most common complication in the first days after hyphema is elevated intraocular pressure. This is usually secondary to outflow obstruction from the red blood cells blocking the trabecular meshwork. However, in some eyes, particularly those with a hyphema at a level above the pupil, pupillary block may cause elevated pressure. In these cases, the pressure can be lowered by merely dilating the pupil.

Corneal blood staining usually occurs where there is a total hyphema in the presence of elevated intraocular pressure for several days. It appears that the pressure must remain over 25 mm Hg for at least 6 days before there is much danger of corneal blood staining. However, blood staining can progress over several hours so that the cornea changes from mildly discolored at a morning examination to opaque the next morning. Therefore, all eyes with total hyphema and with elevated intraocular pressure should have twice-daily slit-lamp examinations, and surgery should be done immediately if any staining is noted.

The most important early complication of traumatic hyphema is secondary hemorrhage. Secondary hemorrhage, or "rebleeding," occurs when the blood clot covering the injured vessel retracts, usually during the 3rd to 5th day after the initial trauma. If the vessel has not healed by this time, rebleeding will occur. There is a secondary hemorrhage in about one third of untreated hyphemas (see "Treatment," below).

Rebleeds worsen the visual prognosis and should be prevented at all costs. It should be emphasized that there is excellent evidence that the initial size of the hyphema cannot be used to predict whether a secondary hemorrhage will occur. A small hyphema, as in this case, should be treated the same as a large hyphema.

Late Complications

Damage to the angle results in chronic glaucoma in 5% to 10% of traumatic hyphemas. The two major sources of damage are angle recession, which occurs at the time of the original injury, and peripheral anterior synechiae, which develop when a hyphema persists for more than about 9 days.

Optic atrophy is thought to occur when the intraocular pressure remains elevated for a prolonged period. Statistically, optic atrophy is unlikely to occur unless the intraocular pressure remains over 50 mm Hg for 5 days or over 35 mm Hg for 7 days. Therefore, surgery to remove a hyphema should be timed so as not to exceed these limits.

Surgery is timed for before the statistical chances of complications become the greatest. Therefore, the ophthalmologist removes the hyphema before

1. The intraocular pressure has remained over 50 mm Hg for 5 days to prevent optic atrophy
2. The intraocular pressure has remained over 35 mm Hg for 7 days to prevent optic atrophy
3. The intraocular pressure has remained over 25 mm Hg for 6 days to prevent corneal blood staining
4. The hyphema has been present for 9 days to prevent formation of peripheral anterior synechiae
5. Corneal blood staining has been present for more than a few hours to prevent staining that may persist for months to years

Treatment

Except under extraordinary circumstances, all children with traumatic hyphema should be admitted to the hospital and permitted restricted or "quiet" activity; in other words, the child is allowed quiet ambulation around the ward with television privileges. Even the best parents cannot ensure that the child will remain quiet at home, and it is not clear whether repeated automobile trips to the doctor increase the chance of rebleeding. In addition, all of the published experience documenting the efficacy of hyphema management has been gleened from hospitalized patients. As well-meaning as the parents may be, it should be explained that the child will have a better chance of visual recovery in the hospital.

Atropine drops, 3 to 4 times daily, should be given to afford examination of the retina, induce cycloplegia for comfort, and prevent pupillary block as previously mentioned. There is no evidence that dilation increases the chance of secondary hemorrhage.

A metal shield should be placed over the involved eye to prevent inadvertent reinjury.

As mentioned earlier, rebleeding occurs when the clot retracts away from an injured vessel that has not fully healed. Antifibrinolytic drugs such as ε-aminocaproic acid delay the retraction of the clot for a few days, thus allowing more time for vessel healing. The use of this drug in a dose of 50 mg/kg/dose every 4 hours up to a maximum of 30 gm/day reduces the chance of rebleeding to under 10%. Common side effects include nausea and vomiting, which is treated with routine antiemetics, and orthostatic hypotension.

If the intraocular pressure is above 25 mm Hg, the full range of pressure-lowering drugs is available. In practice, however, the miotics and epinephrine products are not helpful. Miotics increase inflammation and are likely to induce pupillary block, and the epinephrine drugs do not acutely lower the intraocular pressure. This leaves the β-blockers, the carbonic anhydrase inhibitors, and the osmotics. Practically, timolol, 0.5% twice daily, acetazolamide, 3.5 mg/kg four times daily, and mannitol, 2.5 gm/kg, are appropriate at all ages. Because pupillary block is a contributing factor in many cases of elevated pressure, the pupil should be dilated as previously mentioned, with dilation maintained by atropine.

There is controversy in the literature over the efficacy of topical and systemic steroids in the management of traumatic hyphemas. Topical steroids are occasionally useful when fibrin forms in the anterior chamber, but they do not seem to speed the disappearance of the blood. Some authors have advocated systemic steroids in the prevention of secondary hemorrhage. However, the evidence favoring the use of aminocaproic acid appears to be stronger than that supporting steroids.

In summary, I would admit the child to the hospital, administer aminocaproic acid for the duration of hospitalization, give atropine drops, and monitor the intraocular pressure. If the pressure became elevated, I would use timolol and acetazolamide, if necessary, and would use the aforementioned list to guide any potential surgical intervention. Hospitalization would continue for as long as there is danger of secondary hemorrhage, ordinarily 5 days from the last hemorrhage or rehemorrhage.

Bibliography

1. Palmer DJ, Goldberg MF, Frenkel M, et al: A comparison of two dose regimens of epsilon aminocaproic acid in the prevention and management of secondary traumatic hyphemas. *Ophthalmology* 1986; 93:102–108.
2. Read J, Goldberg MF: Comparison of medical treatment of traumatic hyphema. *Trans Am Acad Ophthalmol Otolaryngol* 1974; 78:799–815.
3. Thomas MA, Parrish RK II, Feuer WJ: Rebleeding after traumatic hyphema. *Arch Ophthalmol* 1986; 104:206–210.

Approach 2

Paul E. Romano, M.D.

Our overall philosophy and approach to the management of primary simple traumatic hyphema in a child (otherwise uncomplicated) is guided by two principles:

First, the most important thing that a physician can do in the management of traumatic hyphema is to prevent the rebleeding episodes. These occur in up to one third of cases. Rebleeding is responsible for almost all of the further complications and bad results that can occur in this condition.

The second principle is therapeutic nihilism. Do the least that one can do that will ensure the desired result. Utilize risk-benefit ratios. Avoid, if at all possible, anything that might make the situation worse.

The best way to minimize the possibility of rebleeding is to give a 5-day course of one of the *systemic* agents that have been shown to reduce the natural rebleeding rate. These include oral steroids (prednisone specifically in childhood), ϵ-aminocaproic acid (Amicar), and tranexamic acid (used in Europe). These agents administered systemically reduce the rebleeding rate to virtually nil (less than 5%). There are many studies in the literature to support the use of these agents. They are approximately equally effective.

We have personally been involved in the management of primary traumatic hyphema[1] treated with systemic steroids in 102 children. There have been only 3 rebleeds, for a rebleed rate of less that 3%. The originator of systemic steroid treatment, Elton Yasuna, M.D., of Boston,[2] has an additional 90 patients without any rebleeds. If you combine all patients who have been treated with systemic (oral) prednisone and reported, both formally and informally, the rebleed rate is 1.56%. In the 3 cases in which rebleeds occurred, they may not be steroid treatment failures at all—in one case the patient did not receive the steroids until almost a day after admission. In the second case, there was manipulation of the eye to remove a subconjunctival BB pellet shortly before rebleed. In the third case the patient was subjected to cervical x-ray films shortly before he rebled. The true rebleed rate with systemic steroid treatment may therefore approach 0%. Similar rebleed rates have been reported with Amicar and tranexamic acid.

We personally prefer steroids because they are considerably cheaper (a 5-day course of Amicar costs close to $200, while a 5-day course of systemic steroids costs about $4). Systemic steroids also have no side effects like nausea, vomiting, muscle cramps, and diarrhea, which affect a significant number of patients taking Amicar. Amicar requires the routine administration of antiemetic drugs. Amicar is specifically contraindicated in sickle cell disease and in pregnancy, while systemic steroids are not. There are almost no contraindications to the use of systemic steroids to halt natural rebleeding in this condition. We use the same dose as Yasuna (prednisone, 0.6 mg/kg/day for 5 days). We don't stop steroid treatment when the blood disappears from the anterior chamber (nor do we discharge the patient from the hospital at that time). At the end of 5 days, treatment with the steroids can be stopped directly. They do not have to be tapered in dosage when administered in these low amounts for this period of time.

Unfortunately, in spite of the overwhelming data published in the literature that support the use of these three systemic drugs, many physicians remain hesitant to treat traumatic hyphema with them. Yet no serious, substantive arguments against them have been raised. To the best of my knowledge, there have been to date no reported or reportable serious or permanent complications from the use of these drugs in this condition. The use of these systemic medications is singularly and by far the most important element of treatment of traumatic hyphema at our current state of knowledge.

We do insist upon 6 days' hospitalization for any child, with bed rest for 5 and bathroom privileges allowed. Others allow "quiet ambulation," which is probably equally effective. To ensure compliance with medication and protect from further injury, this is absolutely necessary for anyone under the age of 18. They are not of an age sufficient to take responsibility for themselves. It is not possible to educate even the best parents to the fearsome complications that often accompany or follow rebleeding episodes. Hospitalization is cost-effective. Over the age of 18, a patient is more likely to understand the significance of his injury or be amenable to listening to an explanation of its dangerous potential. Being of legal age, he is also responsible should he suffer reinjury and a rebleed. We recommend bed rest for 5 days even for adults. But few productive adults will stay at home or in bed for that period of time.

The 7-year-old in this particular case must be hospitalized. We hospitalize the child for a minimum of 6 days: bed rest for 5, up and around on the sixth day prior to going home. Even if the hyphema should be reabsorbed completely prior to 5 days, the patient should not be discharged. Nor should systemic treatment be stopped. The disappearance of blood from the anterior chamber is a good sign but does not ensure against a rebleed. This is a matter of healing and clot dissolution. This is not related to the rate of disappearance of blood from the anterior chamber.

Nor should one take into account the size of the hyphema as to whether the child should be treated and admitted. In the majority of studies there is no correlation whatsoever between rebleeding rate and size of the primary hyphema. In a few studies there are minimal correlations between size of the primary hyphema and the rebleed rate. In the overall picture, therefore, there may be a mild correlation. But, this correlation, if it is present, is so small that it cannot guarantee against a rebleed and cannot be used in any way to direct therapy. Therefore, all hyphemas regardless of size are treated the same way. This patient with a 2-mm hyphema is therefore hospitalized and treated with systemic steroids.

As far as other treatment is concerned, our therapeutic nihilism takes over. Almost all treatment has some risks that must be weighed against possible benefits. The child should wear a perforated shield or some similar vision-permitting, protective device for 5 days. This is to guard against accidental reinjury during this period of greatest tendency to rebleed. Patching (occluding) the eye under the shield for comfort should probably *not* be done. Occlusion of one eye in childhood can result in a strabismus after occlusion for as little as a day or two. Binocular occlusion is not medically indicated. It is contraindicated because of the sensory deprivation and possible psychic trauma.

Also contraindicated in this condition is acute pupillary dilation. This has precipitated rebleeding episodes. We know personally of at least two cases where a rebleeding episode followed shortly after acute dilation at the initial visit. Reed and Goldberg[3] reported similar experiences. Is it really necessary to dilate the pupil to examine the fundus? Rarely are there any traumatic effects to the posterior pole that require immediate, acute, and complete observation and treatment. If you *must* rule out a retinal detachment, we would prefer a gentle B scan echogram. Or atropine may be used. This drug has been studied and does not alter the rebleed rate.

We avoid routine tonometry. We do not treat mild pressure elevations. The eye can tolerate moderately elevated intraocular pressure for several days (50 mm for 5 days, 35 mm Hg for 7 days). Pressure is elevated usually only while there is some blood in the anterior chamber. The pressure is usually not markedly elevated. We advise against routine tonometry, especially in children. In the younger child, it will be a struggle or require sedation. (Admittedly, we know of no case in which a rebleed has been caused by tonometry.) We are, however, concerned with the struggle that may be necessary. If there is evidence of a significant elevation, such as nausea or pain or haziness of the cornea, etc., we would perform tonometry.

We also recommend against the routine use of any glaucoma medications, systemic or topical. We recommend against treatment of mild transient pressure elevations. Miotics irritate the eye and can facilitate pupil block. Virtually all such medications lower the pressure and reduce the tamponade against rebleed. They also reduce the rate of aqueous flow through the anterior chamber. This reduces the rate of clearance of the blood. Blood in the anterior chamber is an irritant. Rebleeding is more likely the more irritated the eye is.

Frequent slit-lamp examination should be performed if there is any concern about corneal blood staining. This is an indication for urgent surgical intervention. It may take several years for a corneal blood stain to disappear. A younger child will get amblyopia and strabismus. Even an adult will likely become strabismic—and ultimately diplopic.

With systemic steroid (oral prednisone) treatment, rebleeding and its feared complications such as blood staining have become so rare that we have not had to perform a surgical treatment or irrigation of a traumatic hyphema for which we have had primary care for over a decade. We have been and continue to be referred cases that do require such treatment. Indications for surgical treatment include, in the case of sickle cell anemia as recommended by Goldberg, an elevated tension of 24 mm Hg for more than a day and the presence of corneal blood staining. Intraocular pressure elevation is not per se an indication for surgical intervention unless it is prolonged for periods of perhaps 4 or 5 days and of a magnitude of 40 or 50 mm Hg or more. If surgery is necessary, we have found trabeculectomy to be the best approach.

For further care, if there is suspicion of damage to the posterior pole of the eye, the pupil may be dilated, preferably with atropine, before sending the patient home. Otherwise, we prefer to postpone the retina examination until 4 to 6 weeks after the initial trauma. At the 6-week visit one should evaluate the angle as well for recession and damage to determine the long-term prognosis and the frequency of follow-up visits. More frequent follow-ups are necessary if there is damage to the angle structure since this increases the possibility of glaucoma later.

In summary, then, the only appropriate treatment for this 7-year-old child requires hospitalization with bed rest for 6 days and treatment with systemic steroids, systemic Amicar, or tranexamic acid. Acute pupillary dilation should be avoided. Atropine should be used if absolutely necessary. Tonometry would not be performed unless there was suspicion of elevated tension. Even if glaucoma is present—if mild (under 40 mm Hg)—because of the transient nature of the glaucoma in this condition, it would not be treated medically. Topical steroids are not a substitute for systemic steroids in this condition. Topical steroids are partially contraindicated because they reduce the rate of clearance of the hyphema. Systemic steroids do not delay the resolution of the hyphema. They do reduce the rebleeding rate to virtually nil. Systemic steroids thereby prevent most of the complications that occur from rebleeding and that are largely responsible for unsuccessful outcomes.

There is a final consideration: the younger the child, the more important is the proper management. We have some evidence that the natural rebleeding rate may, in fact, be highest in the youngest (under 6 years) children (30% to 40%) vs. perhaps only 10% or 15% for older children and adults.

References

1. Rynne MV, Romano PE: Systemic corticosteroids in the treatment of traumatic hyphema. *J Pediatr Ophthalmol Strabismus* 1980; 17:141–143.
2. Yasuna E: Management of traumatic hyphema. *Arch Ophthalmol* 1974; 91:190.
3. Read J, Goldberg MF: Comparison of medical treatment of traumatic hyphema. *Trans Am Acad Ophthalmol Otolaryngol* 1974; 78:799–815.

SECTION V

Retina

Asymptomatic Retinal Breaks—How to Handle the Hole?

APPROACH 1

Norman E. Byer, M.D.

APPROACH 2

Michael J. Elman, M.D.

Case 15 —————————————

Asymptomatic Retinal Breaks— How to Handle the Hole?

A 42-year-old woman is seen for her yearly refraction and ocular examination. Her refraction is $-8.00 =$ 20/20 in each eye. As in the past, the ophthalmologist notes lattice degeneration peripherally, but at this examination a retinal break is noted within the lattice superotemporally in the left eye. No subretinal fluid is present.

Should this break be treated?

Summary

There is little doubt that large retinal detachments should be repaired. However, even retinal specialists continue to debate whether asymptomatic retinal holes should be treated. In this case, a highly myopic woman is discovered to have a retinal hole, and her ophthalmologist must decide whether to treat the area or to observe it.

The conservative approach is advocated by Dr. Byer, who is well respected as an expert in the management of these cases. He reminds us that there is no evidence that treatment is beneficial, but there is quite a bit of natural history data demonstrating the benign nature of atrophic breaks within areas of lattice degeneration.

Dr. Elman stresses the importance of considering other risk factors before deciding on observation of the lesion. In particular, the presence of high myopia in this patient would sway him toward recommending treatment.

The importance of identifying and treating tractional breaks is emphasized by both discussants. This requires careful indirect ophthalmoscopy and, where possible, slit-lamp biomicroscopy.

Approach 1

Norman E. Byer, M.D.

This highly myopic woman in the fifth decade of life with previously known lattice degeneration, which has been managed by observation only, is now found on routine examination to have a retinal break within a superiorly placed lattice lesion. This must therefore be considered an asymptomatic retinal break. The pathogenesis of such breaks within lattice lesions is well known to be on the basis of slowly developing trophic changes and not the result of sudden vitreoretinal traction. Such breaks should more properly be referred to as holes and not tears. They have a high prevalence rate, being found in about 43% of all patients who have lattice degeneration and therefore in approximately 3.4% of persons over the age of 10 years in the general population. Approximately 10% of eyes with lattice combined with atrophic holes eventually collect some subretinal fluid adjacent to one of the holes in a sufficient amount to be termed a *subclinical detachment* according to the definition of Davis (i.e., a detachment extending more than one disc diameter from the hole but no more than two disc diameters posterior to the equator). Even when this happens, they do not require treatment, for 80% to 90% of such small areas of detachment do not progress significantly for many years. Only about 1% to 2% of eyes with lattice and atrophic holes will eventually have a clinical retinal detachment. Also, 50% of such eyes that later have detachment do so prior to the age of 30 years. The absence of any associated subretinal fluid in the present case is a common finding and is consistent with the usually benign course of such lesions. The superotemporal location does not make this break more dangerous. Most retinal detachments associated with this type of break occur in the inferior quadrants. These retinal holes are usually small or tiny (0.1 mm or less in diameter) and are consequently difficult to detect on clinical examination, especially in the absence of subretinal fluid. This is true even with the skillful use of indirect ophthalmoscopy and scleral indentation, which is the best method for detecting them. The usually tiny size plus the absence of symptoms increases the likelihood that this hole may have already been present for a number of years.

It is an interesting observation that among many ophthalmologists there is a rather strong traditional view that such holes in lattice lesions as the one described here are dangerous and should be prophylactically treated. I believe this is because it is really not uncommon to see retinal detachments on this basis, and the conclusion has therefore been drawn that such holes are dangerous. What is very difficult to comprehend is the immense size of the population pool from which such patients come. To illustrate this point, we should realize that around 1 person in 30 over the age of 10 years has both lattice degeneration and at least one hole in one of the lesions. But only about 1% to 2% of these will ever lead to clinical retinal detachment. That is to say, in a population of 3,000 persons over the age of 10 years there will be around 100 with lattice lesions plus round holes, and from this group we may expect only about 1 or 2 with a later clinical retinal detachment. Long-term natural history data confirm their essentially benign course. Therefore prophylactic treatment of the hole in this case presentation would be very ill advised.

The primary danger associated with lattice degeneration is not concerned with the atrophic hole but with the abnormal vitreoretinal traction that exists throughout the fundus, both at the sites of the lattice lesions and also at other sites that cannot be identified prior to the actual onset of tractional retinal tears. Such tears carry a much higher risk, around 35%, of leading to retinal detachment and should be treated promptly with either cryotherapy or possibly argon laser photocoagulation if all lattice lesions can be well visualized with this modality. When this treatment is carried out, it is mandatory that all lattice lesions that can be visualized by the technique of scleral indentation be completely surrounded with treatment.

The refractive status of this patient does not alter the decision that prophylactic treatment is not appropriate. It is still not uncommon to see patients in whom prophylactic treatment has been carried out for such atrophic holes who have then had the unexpected onset of a new tractional retinal tear, with or without a retinal detachment, arising in some other part of the fundus where there may or may not have been a pre-existing lattice lesion. Also, long-term study of fellow eyes has shown that although the risk of detachment increases for lattice in highly myopic eyes, it also increases in the eyes that have received prophylactic treatment, so that this treatment offers no advantage.

This patient would be best managed by occasional observation but not more often than once a year. She should of course be reminded to return for reexamination in the event she experiences retinal symptoms such as light flashes, floaters, loss of side vision, or decreased visual acuity. It is also important to remember that, in discussions with the patient regarding her retinal abnormality, the ophthalmologist should purposely avoid expressing or transmitting apprehension to the patient.

Approach 2 _____

Michael J. Elman, M.D.

The case concerns a highly myopic, apparently asymptomatic woman. On her annual examination, a retinal break is noted within a patch of lattice retinal degeneration superotemporally in her left eye. No subretinal fluid is noted. The history does not indicate whether the retinal break is an atrophic hole or retinal tear. No history is provided on patient activities, previous ocular surgery, or history of trauma. Finally, information on the fellow eye and family history is unavailable.

Indications for Prophylactic Treatment

Fear of retinal detachment underlies the indications for prophylactic treatment in lattice degeneration. However, the risks of progression to retinal detachment must be weighed against the complications and costs of prophylactic treatment. Laser photocoagulation and cryopexy are the preferred methods of treatment. Designed to counteract the forces of vitreoretinal traction exerted on areas of lattice degeneration, these treatments can exacerbate the very forces they are intended to negate. The results may be macular fibroplasia, retinal detachment, or new retinal breaks located adjacent to or 180 degrees opposite the treated area. Therefore, before considering prophylactic treatment, one must analyze fully the risks of a retinal break progressing to detachment. Factors such as family history, refractive status, patient activity, status of the fellow eye, and ocular history must be carefully weighed.

Atrophic Holes

In his landmark work, Byer first questioned the accepted dogma of prophylactic treatment for lattice degeneration and atrophic holes. His recommendation was based on several hundred patients observed safely without treatment for many years. Prior to Byer's report, most retinal surgeons assumed that not treating was dangerous; thus, all patients were treated, which explains the treatment "successes." As in many treatment reports, the best way to "prove" treatment efficacy was to omit proper controls. Without adequate natural history controls, ideally within the context of a well-designed clinical trial, one cannot possibly assess the value of any treatment. Based on Byer's natural history data, the risk of retinal detachment from atrophic holes in lattice degeneration is 0.08%. Before considering prophylactic treatment, one must consider whether other risk factors are present.

Risk Factors

1. Myopia.—Myopic patients harbor a greater risk for retinal detachment. Therefore, myopic eyes with retinal breaks within lattice degeneration warrant prophylactic treatment.

2. Aphakia.—Aphakia increases the risk of retinal detachment tenfold. However, modern methods of cataract extraction (extracapsular cataract extraction with posterior chamber intraocular lens implantation) appear to lessen this risk. Further, breaks tend to appear more frequently in areas of normal retina. While lattice lesions are probably not as important in aphakic detachments as in phakic detachments, breaks within lattice areas may warrant prophylactic treatment in selected aphakic eyes.

3. History of retinal detachment in fellow eye.—Treatment should be strongly considered for eyes with retinal breaks in lattice degeneration when the retina has detached in the fellow eye. We routinely perform such treatment.

4. Family history of retinal detachment.—Prophylactic treatment should be considered for all eyes with lattice degeneration in patients with a family history of retinal detachment. This holds

especially true when the retinal breaks occur in association with lattice lesions.

5. Patient activities.—Active participants in contact sports (i.e., boxing, racquetball, basketball) may warrant prophylactic treatment. At the very least, proper protective eyewear, a polycarbonate lens in a suitably designed frame, should be prescribed. In high-energy contact sports such as hockey or football, eye protection should be integrated into protective headgear. In addition, a propensity for ocular trauma or a history of multiple missed appointment visits may tip the balance in favor of prophylactic treatment vs. observation.

Traction Tears

Traction tears, either within or adjacent to areas of lattice degeneration, should always be treated. The risk for retinal detachment developing in eyes with symptomatic tears ranges between 28% and 35%. As expected, this risk declines to approximately 10% in asymptomatic eyes. Nonetheless, this constitutes a significant risk.

Treatment Methods

The goal of prophylactic treatment is to counterbalance forces of vitreoretinal traction through creation of a chorioretinal scar. Whether using photocoagulation or cryopexy, treatment should never be applied in excess. This will lessen the chances for complications developing. Recent reports suggest that cryopexy may liberate retinal pigment epithelial cells into the vitreous and stimulate the development of proliferative vitreoretinopathy. Nonetheless, cryopexy remains an excellent form of treatment, particularly for extensive or peripheral lesions. As in all ophthalmic procedures, the patient should be made comfortable. Depending on the extent and location of the lesion, either subconjunctival or retrobulbar anesthesia is selected. After treatment, topical corticosteroids and cycloplegic agents are prescribed for 1 week as well as appropriate analgesics. Patients are re-examined 1 month after treatment. They are next seen at 6 months provided no new tears are seen and the treated area shows a nicely pigmented scar at the first postoperative visit.

Examination Frequency

Untreated patients with lattice lesions are examined every 6 to 12 months. All patients, whether treated or untreated, are instructed to return promptly should they undergo severe blunt trauma to the eye or if they experience an increase in flashes or floaters or a decrease in peripheral vision.

Bibliography

1. Byer NE: Review—Lattice degeneration of the retina. *Surv Ophthalmol* 1979; 23:213–247.
2. Davis MD: The natural history of retinal breaks without detachment. *Trans Am Ophthalmol Soc* 1973, 71:343–372.

Diabetic Macular Edema—Focal or Grid Laser?

APPROACH 1

R. Joseph Olk, M.D.

APPROACH 2

Bruce R. Garretson, M.D.

Case 16

Diabetic Macular Edema—Focal or Grid Laser?

A 56-year-old diabetic has had a slowly progressive loss of visual acuity that can be attributed to macular edema. The visual acuity is 20/50 in the right eye and 20/25 in the left. Fluorescein angiography reveals diffuse edema, although there are some areas of lipid surrounding microaneurysms in each eye.

Should either eye be treated, and if so, how?

Summary

Diabetic macular edema is the most common cause of visual loss in diabetics. Unfortunately, until recently this complication of diabetes has not been as extensively studied as the less frequent complication of proliferative retinopathy. However, since 1985 two different techniques have been described that can slow the progression of macular edema and, in some cases, improve the visual acuity. They are the subject of this case discussion.

The technique of "modified grid photocoagulation" was developed and reported by Dr. Olk. In his discussion of this case, Dr. Olk describes this approach, which is aimed at areas of retinal thickening, ischemia, and leakage. The treatment is not simply a grid because he focally treats the leaking areas—hence the term *modified*.

Dr. Garretson describes the indications and techniques developed in the Early Treatment of Diabetic Retinopathy Study (ETDRS). This treatment is primarily aimed at the leaking microaneurysms so common in early diabetic macular edema, and the approach is to ablate each of these "red spots."

It is important to realize that these techniques have different indications: the modified grid is aimed at the problem of diffuse edema, and the ETDRS approach is for focal leakage. Careful patient selection and treatment is necessary if success is to be expected from either method.

Approach 1

R. Joseph Olk, M.D.

For eyes with diffuse diabetic macular edema I recommend modified grid laser photocoagulation treatment.[1,2] Diffuse diabetic macular edema is defined as having two or more disc areas of retinal thickening and involving the center of the macula. Additionally, patients should have a best corrected visual acuity of 20/200 or better and demonstrate no more than 6 clock hours of juxtafoveal capillary nonperfusion on the fluorescein angiogram.

Prior to considering photocoagulation, the patient should be well controlled medically, i.e., the hemoglobin A_{1c} (glycosylated hemoglobin) level equal to or less than 10.0 mg/dL, the patient's diastolic blood pressure less than 100 mm Hg, and no evidence of renal failure. Those patients who are not controlled medically should be referred to their internist for further medical management and asked to return in 3 to 6 months for re-evaluation.

Treatment Technique

The treatment technique is performed as an outpatient procedure, and topical anesthesia is used in almost all cases. If both eyes require treatment, they can be treated consecutively in the same treatment session. A frame of a recent fluorescein angiogram is projected on a Topcon viewer adjacent to the patient to be used as a reference during the treatment session. I use the Mainster posterior pole contact lens.

The argon pure green laser is used to place 100- and 200-μm spots in all areas of diffuse leakage as well as in all areas of capillary nonperfusion as demonstrated on the fluorescein angio-

214

gram. Two to three rows of 100-μm spots are placed up to and including the edge of the foveal avascular zone by spacing the lesions approximately one lesion apart. A similar pattern is utilized for the 200-μm spots at a light intensity with 0.1-second duration. Additional 200-μm spots are usually placed confluently in any areas of obvious focal leakage (Fig 16–1). I would like to emphasize that I believe it is important to try to keep the burns as light as possible, and I try to obtain a burn that is just barely visible at the level of the outer retina or retinal pigment epithelium. The average power settings are 100 to 200 mW, and the average number of spots applied range from 150 to 300 spots per treatment session. The patients are seen every 3 to 4 months, and if clinical examination and/or repeat fluorescein angiogram demonstrate residual retinal thickening, then supplemental modified grid photocoagulation is applied to those areas where residual edema is still present.

It is important to note that, in many instances, modified grid photocoagulation does not need to be applied throughout the entire posterior pole. Again, I emphasize that only those areas of retinal thickening and/or areas of nonperfusion need be treated. Many times this simply involves the retinal areas temporal to the macula (Fig 16–2). In many cases, one can treat the areas of diffuse leakage with a grid pattern and then simply apply additional focal treatment to those areas in the juxtafoveal region that require only focal treatment (Fig 16–3).

If a patient has both macular edema and proliferative diabetic retinopathy, I would recommend the following guidelines: if the patient has "minimal" proliferative retinopathy (i.e., one high-risk characteristic), I would recommend that the macular edema be treated first, to stabilize it and then follow the proliferative disease; panretinal photocoagulation can then be performed at a later time when the proliferative disease progresses. On the other hand, if a patient has "moderate to advanced" proliferative diabetic retinopathy in conjunction with diffuse diabetic macular edema (i.e., two or more high-risk characteristics), then I recommend one of two things: the proliferative disease can be treated first and treatment of the macular edema addressed 3 to 4 months after the proliferative disease has been stabilized. In this instance

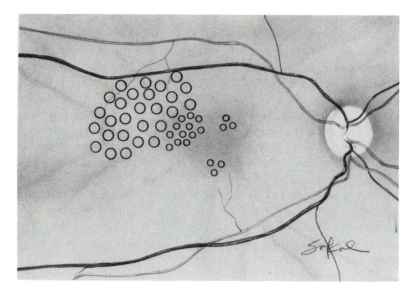

FIG 16–1.
Artist's illustration of modified grid treatment, 2 to 3 rows of 100-μm spots in the juxtafoveal region and 200-μm spots throughout the remaining areas of diffuse leakage and/or nonperfusion. Additional confluent focal treatment was applied to areas of obvious focal leakage. (From Olk RJ: Modified grid argon (blue-green) laser photocoagulation for diffuse diabetic macular edema. *Ophthalmology* 1986; 93:940. Used with permission.)

I would recommend that panretinal photocoagulation *not* be performed in a single session but be performed in two or three sessions because I believe the panretinal photocoagulation in some cases can exacerbate pre-existing macular edema. Alternatively, I have also combined both panretinal photocoagulation and modified grid photocoagulation to the macula in selected cases as well. With this combination, I usually perform the treatment in two or three sessions spaced 2 to 3 weeks apart. At the first session one third to one half of the peripheral inferior part of the retina is treated with panretinal photocoagulation, and modified grid photocoagulation for the diffuse macular edema is applied to the affected areas. The patient is then scheduled to return for one or two supplemental panretinal photocoagulation treatments, after which we wait approximately 3 months and reassess the situation. If there is residual macular edema, supplemental modified grid photocoagulation is applied, and if residual proliferative disease requiring additional panretinal treatment is also indicated, I will apply it at the same time.

Most patients with diffuse diabetic macular edema require two or more modified grid treatments.

Side Effects

Most patients who undergo modified grid laser photocoagulation complain of paracentral scotomas. These tend to diminish with time but never completely disappear. Patients should be advised of this side effect preoperatively.

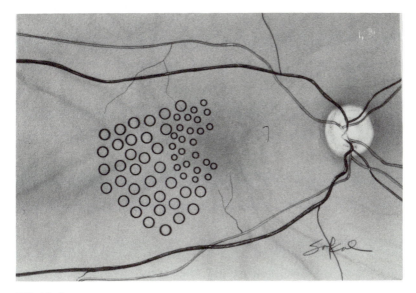

FIG 16–2.
Artist's illustration of modified grid treatment, 100- and 200-μm spots applied to the temporal macular area and area of diffuse leakage and/or nonperfusion. (From Olk RJ: Modified grid argon (blue-green) laser photocoagulation for diffuse diabetic macular edema. *Ophthalmology* 1986; 93:940. Used with permission.)

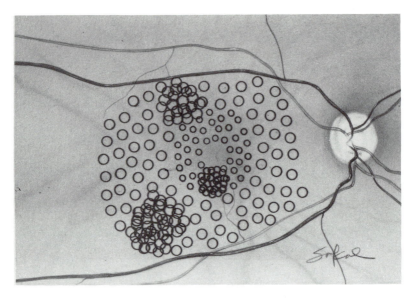

FIG 16–3.
Artist's illustration of modified grid treatment, 100- and 200-μm spots applied to area of diffuse leakage and/or nonperfusion superotemporal to the macula; additional focal areas were treated nasally and inferior to the foveal vascular zone. (From Olk RJ: Modified grid argon (blue-green) laser photocoagulation for diffuse macular edema. *Ophthalmology* 1986; 93:940. Used with permission.)

Case Examples

Case 1

Case 1 (Fig 16–4), a 56-year-old type II (non–insulin-dependent) diabetic of 26 years' duration, demonstrates diffuse macular edema temporal to the foveal avascular zone with early central cystoid formation. The visual acuity was 20/40 (Fig 16–4,A and B). A modified grid was applied to the entire area of diffuse leakage (Fig 16–4,C). Three months later, the central cystoid has cleared, and visual acuity has improved to 20/25 (Fig 16–4,D and E).

Case 2

Case 2 (Fig 16–5), a 50-year-old type II (non–insulin-dependent) diabetic of 1 year's duration, had received panretinal pho-

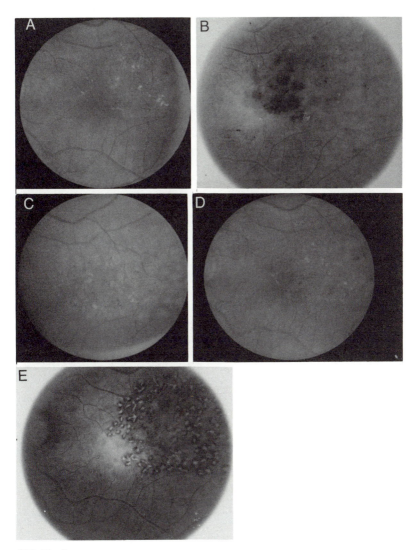

FIG 16–4.
A–E, case 1. See text.

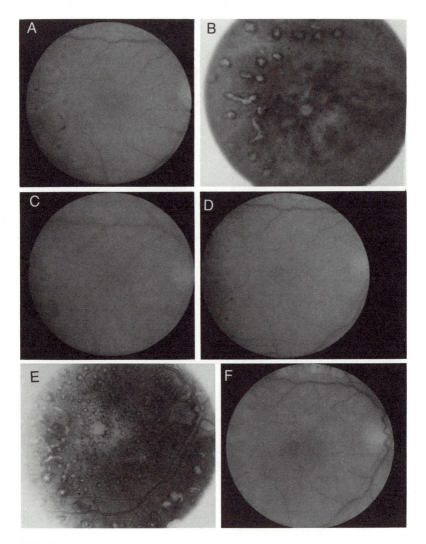

FIG 16–5.
A–E, case 2. See text.

tocoagulation 6 months prior. Diffuse diabetic macular edema was present, with visual acuity reduced to 20/40 (Fig 16–5,A and B). A modified grid was applied throughout the posterior pole to all areas of diffuse leakage (Fig 16–5,C). Four months later, the visual acuity was 20/32, and the macular edema had resolved (Fig 16–5,D and E). One year post-treatment the vision remained 20/32 (Fig 16–5,F).

Case 3

Case 3 (Fig 16–6), a 41-year-old type I insulin-dependent diabetic of 16 years' duration, had been given focal treatment temporal to the macula 5 years prior. Examination reveals severe neovascularization elsewhere (NVE) and vitreous hemorrhage (three high-risk characteristics) and diffuse macular edema with intraretinal cystoid formation. The visual acuity was 20/40 (Fig 16–6,A and B). Modified grid photocoagulation was applied in conjunction with panretinal photocoagulation to the inferior half of the peripheral fundus (Fig 16–6,C and D). Three weeks later the superior half of the peripheral retina was treated with panretinal photocoagulation (Fig 16–6,E and F). One year post-treatment the macular edema had resolved, and the visual acuity stabilized at 20/40 (Fig 16–6,G and H).

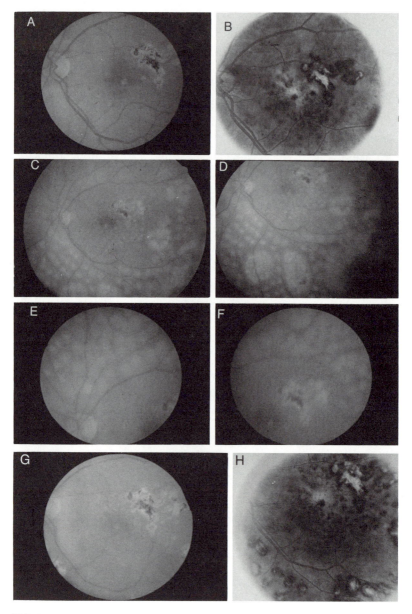

FIG 16–6.
A–H, case 3. See text.

References

1. Olk RJ: Modified grid argon (blue-green) laser photocoagulation for diffuse diabetic macular edema. *Ophthalmology* 1986; 93:938–950.
2. Olk RJ: Argon green versus krypton red modified grid laser photocoagulation for diffuse diabetic macular edema—A preliminary report, in *Second International Laser Symposium.* 1987, in press.

Approach 2

Bruce R. Garretson, M.D.

Macular edema is the most common cause of visual handicap in diabetics today. The case presented is typical of this large group of patients in that the patient has experienced a slowly progressive decline in the central visual acuity of both eyes.

Until recently, the rationale for treatment and hope for improvement in these patients has been limited. In 1985, the ETDRS research group published results of a multicentered randomized clinical trial of argon laser photocoagulation for patients with "clinically significant" macular edema.[1, 2] The study included a broad range of patients with variable degrees of diabetic maculopathy. Clinically significant macular edema included any or all the following:

1. Retinal thickening involving or within 500 μm of the center of the macula
2. Hard exudate(s) at or within 500 μm of the center of the macula if associated with thickening of adjacent retina (but not residual hard exudates remaining after disappearance of retinal thickening)
3. A zone or zones of retinal thickening one disc area or larger in size, any part of which is within one disc diameter of the center of the macula

After 3 years of follow-up, 12% of eyes in the treatment group experienced significant visual loss (at least a doubling of the initial visual angle) as compared with 24% of eyes in the untreated group. On this basis, it was recommended that treatment be considered in all diabetics with clinically significant macular edema, although the decision of whether and when to treat must be individualized for each patient. Once the decision to treat is made, controversy remains in the decision of what type of treatment to offer, i.e., focal ablation, diffuse grid pattern, or combined treatment.

Our patient has diffuse edema in both eyes with scattered microaneurysms and exudates. Visual acuity is 20/50 OD and 20/25 OS, with clear media and no evidence of proliferative retinopathy. Utilizing the ETDRS criteria, I believe that focal argon laser treatment of the right eye should be offered to this patient. Although the left eye also meets our treatment criteria, I generally do not treat eyes with visual acuities of 20/30 or better unless there is a discrete leaking focus with a surrounding circinate lipid ring threatening the fovea or there has been documented progression of the macular edema. Many patients with good visual acuity and macular edema complain bitterly of paracentral scotomas after treatment, although the subjective awareness of these defects tends to lessen with time.

Treatment Regimen

Intravenous fluorescein angiography is generally performed prior to treatment in order to demonstrate treatable lesions within two disc diameters of the center of the foveal avascular zone. Treatable lesions are identified as discrete points of retinal hyperfluorescence and focal leakage greater than 300 μm from the center of the fovea. I avoid treating retinal hemorrhages larger than 100 μm that are unassociated with leakage. In cooperative patients, topical anesthesia alone is generally adequate.

Using an argon green laser, one should attempt to blanch or whiten each individual microaneurysm and areas of leakage within a treatment area. Typical laser spot size ranges from 50 to 100 μm, although a 50-μm spot size is recommended for areas of leakage from 300 to 500 μm from the center of the foveal avascular zone. Also, it is important to use a short duration of 0.1 seconds or less in order to minimize spread of the burn. I use the minimum power necessary to produce the desired effect and usually begin at 150 mW of power. At the completion of the treatment it is necessary to reinspect the treated lesions because some of the microaneurysms will become reperfused and require additional treatment. I generally re-examine my patients 3 to 4 months after laser treatment. Best corrected visual acuity is obtained, and fluorescein angiography is performed at this visit. Retreatment is indicated if persistent areas of focal leakage causing clinically significant macular edema remain.

In all diabetics, normalization of blood glucose levels is desirable. A recent prospective study comparing a group of type I diabetic patients with tight glucose regulation utilizing continuous subcutaneous insulin pumps with a group of patients receiving conventional insulin therapy demonstrated a slowing in the progression of early diabetic retinopathy in the group with better glycemic control.[3] The clinical significance of this intensive glycemic regulation is unknown, and strong evidence regarding the therapeutic benefit of tight glucose control on the development and progression of macular edema is lacking. The ETDRS is also investigating the use of aspirin in diabetic patients in a randomized manner with respect to the development of diabetic retinopathy. To date a significant effect on the retinopathy has not been reported.

References

1. Early Treatment Diabetic Retinopathy Study Research Group: Photocoagulation for diabetic macular edema. Early treatment diabetic retinopathy study report #1. *Arch Ophthalmol* 1985; 103:1796–1806.
2. Early Treatment Diabetic Retinopathy Study Research Group: Treatment techniques and clinical guidelines for photocoagulation of diabetic macular edema. Early treatment diabetic retinopathy study report #2. *Ophthalmology* 1987; 94:761–774.
3. Rosenstock J, Friberg T, Raskin P: Effect of glycemic control on microvascular complications in patients with type 1 diabetes mellitus. *Am J Med* 1986; 81:1012–1018.

Central Serous Chorioretinopathy— The If's and When's of Treatment

APPROACH 1

Lawrence A. Yannuzzi, M.D.

APPROACH 2

Howard Schatz, M.D.

Case 17 _____

Central Serous Chorioretinopathy—The If's and When's of Treatment

A 36-year-old physician complains of blurred vision in the left eye. Examination reveals a visual acuity of 20/40, metamorphopsia, and an area of elevation in the fundus near the fovea. A fluorescein angiogram reveals an area of central serous chorioretinopathy one disc diameter from the fovea.

What treatment, if any, should be offered?

Summary

Central serous chorioretinopathy is a condition that affects those individuals who need their vision the most: young, busy professionals. As in this case, most ophthalmologists have physicians in their practices with central serous chorioretinopathy. There is significant debate about when these lesions should be treated, if ever. Two experts in the treatment of retinal disease discuss that question in terms of this case.

Dr. Yannuzzi tends toward the approach that a patient, unless extremely distressed by metamorphopsia, should be followed for at least 3 months after the first attack before considering treatment. He emphasizes the complications of treatment.

In his discussion, Dr. Schatz states that if he were in this patient's place he would prefer to have immediate treatment because that would reduce the time to resolution of his metamorphopsia. Clearly, this would be a fully informed decision!

Both of these authors stress the importance of avoiding treatment within one-half disc diameter of the center of the fovea. This is a danger zone in which the risk of complications far outweighs the potential benefit in almost all cases.

Approach 1 _____

Lawrence A. Yannuzzi, M.D.

In this 36-year-old physician who is presumably a male and white (at least according to the profile in our practice), the visual symptoms are consistent with an exudative detachment of his macula. This is also evidently the first episode of visual dysfunction since there was no history of a previous complaint.

The angiogram revealed a focal leak that was not suspicious of a vascular phenomenon, specifically choroidal neovascularization. This suggests the diagnosis of central serous chorioretinopathy. Decisions regarding management require an understanding of the natural course of the disease.

Natural Course

There is no definitive study on the natural course of this disease. However, most studies have indicated that the primary detachment will resolve spontaneously in more than 80% of the eyes in 3 to 4 months. Recurrences are the rule, although there is a tremendous variability. The visual prognosis, most would agree, is also fairly good in the primary attack. With recurrent detachments, the risk for perifoveal atrophy and cystic degeneration with associated visual decline increases, as one would expect. The same risks exist with a detachment of long duration but, curiously, some patients have recurrent bouts, and others have solitary episodes with prolonged detachment and no visual decline.

Medical Therapy

In general, there is no place for medical therapy in this disease. It is clear that many of the patients have so-called type A personalities. However, we do not suggest behavioral intervention therapy in a patient even if there is an obvious type A behavioral character. We do stress the possible relationship between a sympathetic response and this disease and urge the patient to assume a more mild temperament and life-style. This would be particularly relevant to a physician who could understand the relationship between circulating adrenergic factors and the presence of catecholamine receptors at the level of the pigment epithelium.

Other medical treatments that have been advocated in the past, such as corticosteroids, may actually be associated with recurrent attacks in some patients.

At this point in our discussion with the patient, we would explain the nature of the condition and review the demographic features, the known information regarding its natural course, and some of the concepts regarding its pathogenesis. We could then discuss laser therapy.

Laser Treatment

It is important to realize that there is no absolute clinical trial that supports the efficacy and safety of laser photocoagulation treatment. There are one or two studies that suggest that there is a tendency for reduced recurrences but no visual stabilization or improvement with treatment. On the basis of our current understanding of the condition, I would only consider the following patients for treatment:

1. A patient who has a primary detachment that persists for longer than 3 months and who has a pigment epithelial leak that is remote from the center of the fovea (one-half disc diameter or greater).

2. A patient who has a detachment that persists for 6 months or longer with associated visual decline and a leak that is close to the center of the fovea.

3. A patient who has demonstrated severe vision loss in one eye from the condition and has developed a primary detachment in the fellow eye. In such a patient, I would consider earlier intervention since it is known that photocoagulation does reduce the duration of the detachment.

4. A patient who has had recurrent detachments and progressive visual decline. I would try to reduce the duration of the detachment in this patient with photocoagulation therapy at an earlier point in his course.

5. A patient who has severe visual discomfort from the metamorphopsia. This patient must be willing to accept the scotoma associated with photocoagulation as a substitute for the metamorphopsia. I might add that I *very rarely* see a patient like this since a very detailed explanation of the risks, limitations, and potential benefits of photocoagulation treatment usually results in the patient being more willing to accept the metamorphopsia.

6. A darkly pigmented individual with central serous chorioretinopathy. Although it is my impression that patients who tend to be more pigmented seem to have earlier decompensation of the pigment epithelium with visual decline, these patients are not at as much risk for disciform disease (iatrogenically induced by photocoagulation) than are their white counterparts. This is an unproven observation that may be a function of more pronounced contrast at the level of the pigment epithelium in darkly pigmented individuals when atrophy is first evolving. I do not think it matters what wavelength is used for photocoagulation. Krypton red works as well as argon pure green. I would not use the argon blue light because of its phototoxicity.

7. A patient with a dependent inferior detachment secondary to a macular retinal pigment epithelial (RPE) leak or leaks.

8. A patient with the variant of central serous chorioretinopathy: serous bullous detachment with multiple RPE detachments and active RPE leaks.

While the aforementioned points are relative indications for treatment, most patients should not be treated. Since there is no known visual benefit in treating cases compared with controls, it is hard to justify treatment in most patients. I do not use recurrence as an indicator for treatment since numerous patients have multiple recurrences without developing significant pigment epithelial degenerations or cystic degeneration of the macula with visual decline. In addition, there are real potential complications that must be considered.

Complications of Therapy

1. In juxtafoveal leaks, there is the possibility of postphotocoagulation disruption of Bruch's membrane, and choroidal neovascularization may follow. In addition, we must keep in mind that photocoagulation of such juxtafoveal leaks converts metamorphopsia to a scotoma, which is more troublesome to some patients.

2. Inadvertent damage to the fovea or other nonpathological tissue or an inadvertent macular hole from intense photovaporization (usually associated with a small spot size and a short burst of intense energy) may occur. This also can stimulate choroidal neovascularization and elicit a disciform process.

Finally, I think it is important for patients to monitor their vision carefully with self-assessment testing utilizing the Amsler grid or the Yannuzzi card. Bilateral manifestations are frequent with respect to essentially nonexudative changes and less common with respect to bilateral detachments.

Approach 2 _____

Howard Schatz, M.D.

In this case of a 36-year-old physician with 20/40 vision due to central serous chorioretinopathy, if the leak were nearer the fovea than a one-half disc diameter, I would not recommend treatment. It has been shown that when a leak is within a half disc diameter from the center of the fovea the risk of a complication is highly significant. The risks of treating close leaks are development of subretinal neovascularization at the treatment-leak site, hitting the fovea, and causing a scar. It is not worth treating close leaks unless there is some unusual, very compelling circumstance.

When a leak is more than a half disc diameter from the center of the fovea, as in this case, I think the patient should be given the opportunity to make the decision as to treatment or no treatment. We know that treatment shortens the course, that is, shortens the duration of the condition. Treatment has not been proved to result in better visual acuity in the long run. Some patients do not need to have excellent central vision in each eye and can live very comfortably for a few months with a sensory detachment of the macula. Other patients may find it very difficult to do their work. An ophthalmologist, for instance, would have a very hard time doing surgery and examining patients if there was a sensory detachment in one eye. I, personally, have thought about this problem for myself if the situation ever arose that I developed central serous chorioretinopathy. I would want to have treatment immediately, within a day or two of the discovery of a sensory detachment and a pigment epithelial leak, if it were more than a half disc diameter from the central fovea.

So, when a leak is more than a half disc diameter from the

center of the fovea, I do tell patients about the two alternatives: treatment or no treatment. I go through the pros and cons and risks and hazards of each. I think in experienced hands the treatment of a leak far from the fovea carries with it an extremely small risk and is certainly legitimate in patients who understand the issues and have the need for good central visual acuity in each eye.

One final note: There is a condition called chronic severe recurrent central serous chorioretinopathy. In this condition patients have had many leaks, the leaks are chronic, and the patients have severe changes of the pigment epithelium with field defects. In such patients when a leak arises, it is probably best to treat soon rather than allow the patient to have subretinal fluid for long periods of time because their retina is already severely damaged and it is possible that more chronic fluid would cause more permanent, irreversible damage. Such are special cases, somewhat unusual, but in such cases treatment should be done earlier than not.

Bibliography

1. Schatz H, Yannuzzi LA, Gitter KA: Subretinal neovascularization following argon laser photocoagulation treatment for central serous chorioretinopathy: Complications or misdiagnosis. *Trans Am Acad Ophthalmol Otolaryngol* 1977; 83:893–906.

Neuro-ophthalmology

Case 18

Transient Visual Loss— What Kind of Workup?

APPROACH 1

Stephen C. Pollock, M.D.

APPROACH 2

Peter J. Savino, M.D.

Case 18 _____

Transient Visual Loss—What Kind of Workup? _____

At the time of a routine refraction, a 62-year-old woman relates several episodes of sudden blurring of her vision during a 2-week period, each lasting several minutes. She cannot remember whether it occurred in one or both eyes. She is not terribly concerned about these attacks but wonders if they "mean anything."

Should these be investigated?

Summary _____

This patient, as often happens, relates transient visual symptoms during an otherwise routine visit. The ophthalmologist must decide whether the symptoms warrant further investigation or whether they should be ignored.

Dr. Pollock stresses the importance of obtaining historical information, not only of the episodes themselves but also of any other systemic abnormalities that could give a clue to the etiology of the symptoms.

Dr. Savino also notes the importance of the history, especially as it relates to whether the visual loss was monocular, binocular, or homonymous. If the patient is not certain of the location of the visual symptoms, they should be assumed to be bilateral, which implicates the vertebrobasilar circulation.

The important point in both of these discussions is that any transient visual loss should be investigated, at least by using simple techniques such as history, ocular examination, and probably evaluation by an internist who has an understanding of the various etiologies that could be involved.

Approach 1 _____

Stephen C. Pollock, M.D.

Stroke remains an important cause of serious morbidity and mortality in this country. Only rarely do strokes occur without warning; most are preceded by symptoms indicative of transient cerebral or ocular ischemia. Conversely, patients who experience transient focal neurological symptoms (transient ischemic attacks [TIAs]) are recognized to be at increased risk for the subsequent development of stroke. Visual loss is the sole symptom or the predominant symptom in a large percentage of TIAs and is strongly correlated with the presence of atheromatous disease involving the carotid or vertebrobasilar circulations. In addition, a number of disease processes other than atherosclerosis can lead to transient visual loss. In the evaluation of patients with episodic visual symptoms, it is essential to identify those who have an increased risk of stroke due to treatable disease so that appropriate therapeutic measures can be undertaken without delay.

Patients who experience transient visual disturbances from any cause often obtain ophthalmologic consultation, and not surprisingly, ophthalmologists are frequently the first physicians to evaluate such patients. Even so, the problem of transient visual loss can be a source of uncertainty for many ophthalmologists. There are several reasons for this. First, the ephemeral nature of the symptoms and the fact that successive episodes may be separated by a symptom-free interval lasting weeks or even months nearly always precludes an opportunity to examine the patient when symptoms are present. Consequently, the physician must relay on historical information, which may be vague, and on circumstantial clinical signs to formulate an initial clinical impression. A second cause of uneasiness is the recognition that transient visual disturbances often reflect underlying nonocular disease, the management of which does not fall exclusively within the purview of the ophthalmologist. Finally, the literature on existing diagnostic and therapeutic modalities, though voluminous, is nevertheless inconclusive with regard to a number of important issues and is frequently contradictory. However, despite the imperfect state of our knowledge, I believe that a rational approach to the patient with transient visual loss is possible and that the ophthalmologist, by virtue of frequent early contact with such patients, skill in specialized examination techniques, and a comprehensive understanding of the visual system, is in a unique position to initiate the diagnostic evaluation and, in many cases, to impact favorably on the patient's prognosis.

At the outset, it is important to draw a distinction between what should be done for the patient and what the extent of the ophthalmologist's involvement ought to be. Certain management decisions will necessarily be made by neurologists, cardiologists, vascular surgeons, etc., either alone or in concert with the referring ophthalmologist. In my view, the ophthalmologist's obligations are as follows: (1) recognize transient visual symptoms as possibly indicative of serious underlying disease, (2) acquire as much relevant data from the history and physical examination as possible in order to narrow the differential diagnosis, and (3) make *timely* referrals to the appropriate colleagues when indicated. The ophthalmologist's role in treatment of the patient's disorder will depend in large part on the diagnosis.

Symptoms related to ischemia typically have an abrupt onset. The visual disturbances considered here likewise begin precipitously and terminate just as quickly or nearly so. With few exceptions, they result from a temporary interruption of the blood flow to the eye or to a portion of the brain, usually the visual cortex. To qualify as "transient," the symptoms must resolve within 30 minutes of their onset. Though somewhat arbitrary, this requirement effectively differentiates visual symptoms having a vascular origin from those arising from several common ocular disorders (early corneal edema, certain ocular surface abnormalities, and fluctuations in the refractive state of the eye that result from changes in serum osmolarity). Temporary regional reduction of blood flow may result from several pathophysiological mechanisms including vasospasm, vasculitis, systemic hypotension, compression of blood vessels, and thromboembolism. These mechanisms and the diseases with which they are associated should be kept in mind when acquiring and analyzing clinical data. Thromboembolic disease, in particular, must always be considered when evaluating a patient with transient visual loss.

With regard to the evaluation and management of patients with transient disturbances of vision, the following guidelines and recommendations are offered.

History

Several key pieces of historical information will help to place the patient in one or another of the major diagnostic categories.

Try to determine whether the symptoms are monocular or binocular. Transient monocular visual loss, termed *amaurosis fugax*, occurs when the blood supply to the eye or optic nerve is compromised on the affected side. Thromboembolic disease of the anterior circulation is an important cause (though certainly not the only one) and should always be considered when monocular visual loss is reported. Binocular visual disturbances may involve the entire field in each eye or may be confined to a portion of the field, in which case the perceived defects are homonymous. In general, binocular defects are due to ischemia of the visual cortex and thus imply reduced blood flow within the vertebrobasilar system. Less commonly, transient homonymous defects accompany temporary hemodynamic disturbances in the disc distribution of the middle cerebral artery. Keep in mind that patients with homonymous visual loss may not be aware of the binocular nature of their symptoms and will unwittingly localize the problem to the eye on the hemianopic side. When a patient is unsure as to whether symptoms occurred in one or both eyes, as in the case presented here, monocular involvement must be viewed as a distinct possibility, and the diagnostic evaluation should be conducted accordingly.

Inquire about the duration of visual symptoms. Visual loss

consistent with amaurosis fugax typically lasts one to several minutes. By contrast, the episodic blink-outs described by patients with papilledema or optic disc drusen are fleeting and last no more than a second or two. Note that from a practical standpoint the diagnosis of papilledema or disc drusen is based primarily on the examination, not on the history.

Identify any precipitants. Visual loss brought on by standing implicates orthostatic hypotension and also suggests that the circulation to the affected part of the visual system is already compromised even under optimal conditions. Transient binocular visual loss with changes in head position suggests vertebrobasilar insufficiency. Sudden visual loss in one eye that consistently occurs with eccentric gaze and then resolves when the eyes are brought back into the primary position is termed *gaze-evoked amaurosis*. Patients with this complaint are very likely to be harboring an intraorbital tumor on the affected side, usually a meningioma or hemangioma.

Document any associated symptoms. The concurrence of visual loss and one or more symptoms of brain stem ischemia (diplopia, disequilibrium, vertigo, dysarthria, dysphagia, perioral numbness, or sudden weakness of the legs) points to vertebrobasilar insufficiency, either from atheromatous thromboembolism involving the posterior circulation or from cardiac emboli. Hemispheric symptoms such as aphasia or hemiparesis, on the other hand, should lead the examiner to suspect emboli of carotid origin or, much less commonly, cardiac origin. Visual symptoms preceded by angina or palpitations are most likely due to cardiac emboli, as are multifocal symptoms.

Migraine aura is a very common cause of recurrent stereotyped disturbances of vision. The hallmark of migrainous visual loss is the perception of scintillations—visual hallucinations that take the form of flickering lights, zig-zag lines, sparkles, or stars. Colors and geometric shapes have been described as well. When scintillations are present, the symptoms are always binocular and begin within discreet homonymous portions of the visual field. Typically, the hallucination enlarges, moves across the visual field, and disappears after 15 to 20 minutes. The involved portions of the field remain scotomatous for a short period of time after the scintillations have dissipated. The subsequent development of a throbbing headache supports the diagnosis of migraine, but headache may be absent in a patient with an otherwise typical migraine symptom complex ("acephalgic migraine"). A positive family history of migraine lends weight to the diagnosis as well. Vasospasm involving the ophthalmic or retinal circulations can produce monocular visual loss without scintillations or headache that is indistinguishable from amaurosis fugax. Termed *ocular migraine,* it is always a diagnosis of exclusion.

Be certain to document the presence or absence of the major recognized risk factors for vascular disease and stroke: high blood pressure, diabetes, hypercholesterolemia, previous stroke or TIA, cardiac disease (myocardial infarction, congestive heart failure, arrhythmia, rheumatic fever, prosthetic valves), smoking, use of birth control pills, and a family history of cerebrovascular or cardiac disease. This information provides a clinical context in which to judge the a priori likelihood of there being an underlying vasculopathologic process.

Complaints of unilateral ocular pain should prompt consideration of ocular ischemia from ipsilateral carotid artery stenosis or occlusion. Similarly, angina and calf claudication suggest the presence of atherosclerotic vascular disease. Elderly patients should be questioned about symptoms of temporal arteritis. In young or middle-aged patients, symptoms related to systemic lupus or other autoimmune vasculitides should be reviewed. Constitutional symptoms may accompany a number of diseases associated with transient visual loss including hyperviscosity syndromes, infective endocarditis, cardiac myxoma, and virtually any form of vasculitis and should be addressed routinely.

Examination

The examiner should specifically look for the ocular manifestations of carotid insufficiency and for evidence of previous embolic events. The association between peripheral retinal blot hemorrhages and ipsilateral occlusive disease of the internal carotid artery is well established. Less well known is the fact that carotid artery disease is the third most common cause of rubeosis of the iris and angle behind diabetes and central retinal vein occlusion. Advanced rubeosis with *low* intraocular pressure (presumably due to hyposecretion of the ciliary body) is virtually pathognomonic of profoundly reduced blood flow through the carotid and/or ophthalmic arteries. Signs of anterior segment ischemia may occur as well. The finding of intravascular retinal emboli unequivocally signals the presence of an embolic source in the heart or carotid system. Although opinions may differ, I tend to believe that the site of origin of these emboli can often be determined on the basis of their ophthalmoscopic appearance. The yellow or copper-colored refractile plaques situated at arteriolar bifurcations represent cholesterol emboli from an ulcerated lesion in the carotid artery. Less commonly observed are the chalk-white concretions found in vessels on or near the optic disc that are particles of calcium dislodged from diseased heart valves. Platelet-fibrin thrombi are gray-white and evanescent and are rarely seen. Although cholesterol plaques per se probably do not cause symptoms—they rarely obstruct blood flow in the retina—their occurrence in a patient with amaurosis fugax confirms the presence of atheromatous disease of the carotid artery and indicates that the patient is at increased risk for both stroke and death. A complete neurovascular examination additionally includes auscultation and palpation of the cervical carotid arteries and measurement of retinal artery perfusion pressure. For the latter, I prefer ophthalmodynamometry because it is safe, quick, and simple to perform. Findings predictive of arterial disease include a carotid bruit, reduced carotid artery pulsations, and reduced retinal artery pressure. Carotid palpation carries a very small but definite risk of precipitating a cerebral ischemic event and may reasonably be omitted by the ophthalmologist. Comparison of the ophthalmodynamometry value obtained in one eye with that obtained in the other is probably more meaningful for diagnostic purposes than comparison of these values against a normal standard.

Ancillary Studies

A complete blood count, erythrocyte sedimentation rate, and determination of serum glucose, serum cholesterol, and triglyceride levels should be ordered routinely. In addition, all patients with transient visual symptoms should have electrocardiography (ECG) performed. Depending on the clinical context, the following investigations may be indicated as well: antinuclear antibody and other tests for autoimmune vasculitis, serum protein electrophoresis, cryoglobulin levels, chest x-ray, temporal artery biopsy, and computed tomography (CT) scan of the head and orbits.

Echocardiogram

A cardiac source of emboli should be considered in all patients who complain of transient visual loss. M-mode and 2-dimensional echocardiography is a safe, noninvasive means for detecting structural abnormalities of the heart. Among patients with symptoms of cerebral or ocular ischemia, it is most likely to provide clinically significant information in patients under the age of 45, patients with prosthetic heart valves or a history of rheumatic heart disease, patients suspected of having a cardiac myxoma or infective endocarditis, and those with multifocal symptoms. The majority of elderly individuals with transient visual loss will be found to have evidence of arterial disease. By contrast, the incidence of cardiac lesions capable of shedding emboli is quite low, which makes it unlikely that a significant cardiac lesion will be detected by echocardiography. Nevertheless, the fact that the rest is risk free justifies its use even when the anticipated yield of useful information is relatively low. It should certainly be performed prior to angiography in older patients who are being considered for carotid endarterectomy, especially if neurovascular examination findings are normal or there is a history of cardiac disease. In patients of any age, if the cardiac examination and ECG show normal function, it is unlikely that an echocardiogram will disclose pathology.

Noninvasive Studies

Awareness of the inherent dangers and limitations of carotid angiography has spawned a bewildering array of diverse techniques for measuring blood flow in the carotid or ophthalmic circulations and for imaging lesions of the cervical carotid artery. These tests can be used to confirm suspected atheromatous involvement of the carotid system in patients with transient visual loss and evidence of atherosclerosis by history and examination and to exclude the presence of a lesion in symptomatic patients who have a low a priori risk of atherosclerotic disease, particularly those under 40 years of age. The most widely used tests are Doppler ultrasound and B-mode ultrasound. They provide complimentary information about blood flow and vessel contour and may be employed in combination (a "duplex" scan). Unfortunately, neither modality is 100% sensitive for detecting carotid lesions, and neither provides information about the carotid siphon or intracranial circulation. Thus, they do not obviate the need for angiography in symptomatic patients who are considered possible surgical candidates. However, because they are noninvasive, both tests may be performed serially to detect progression of atheromatous lesions. In addition, B-mode ultrasound affords direct visualization of the vessel wall and can provide more information about the nature of an ulcerative or stenotic lesion than can be obtained with angiography. These techniques may eventually lead to more precise correlations between clinical parameters and stroke risk and should help to define which subgroups of patients will benefit from surgery.

Angiogram

Among carotid studies, intra-arterial angiography represents the "gold standard." It is performed in patients with monocular transient visual loss or hemispheric TIA to detect surgically amenable lesions of the extracranial carotid artery and to evaluate the intracranial circulation. The procedure is associated with a small but definite risk of stroke or death. With few exceptions, it should not be performed in patients who, for medical or other reasons, are not suitable candidates for surgery.

Management
General Measures

Control of hypertension, cessation of smoking, and normalization of serum cholesterol levels are important aspects of stroke prevention in all patients and are best managed by an internist.

Admission to the Hospital

The decision whether or not to admit a patient who complains of transient visual loss ordinarily is based on the amount of time that has elapsed since the onset of symptoms. Although reliable data on the natural history of untreated amaurosis fugax is not currently available, it is known that the risk of stroke following TIA is greatest within the first month after the onset of symptoms. It seems reasonable to presume that patients who complain of recent-onset (less than 2 months) amaurosis have an increased risk of stroke compared with patients whose symptoms are similar except that they have been present for a longer period of time. Consideration should be given to admitting such patients under the care of an internist or neurologist, both to expedite the diagnostic evaluation and to facilitate instituting anticoagulation therapy should this be indicated. With regard to admission, a recent increase in the frequency of episodes should be considered the equivalent of new-onset symptoms.

Pharmacological Therapy

Options include antiplatelet therapy and anticoagulation.

Antiplatelet Therapy

Several prospective clinical trials have demonstrated that aspirin, 650 mg twice daily, reduces the incidence of stroke in patients with TIA. There is recent evidence that much lower doses (350 mg daily or less) have the same prophylactic value but with fewer side effects. One aspirin per day is indicated in the following settings: (1) binocular transient visual loss in patients with evidence of atherosclerosis whose symptoms are felt to represent vertebrobasilar insufficiency and (2) monocular symptoms associated with an ipsilateral carotid artery lesion in patients who are poor medical risks for surgery or who are found to have angiographic contraindications to endarterectomy. Aspirin may also have a beneficial effect in patients with recurrent symptoms but no evidence of atherosclerosis; such patients are typically under 40 years of age.

Anticoagulation

Warfarin has been used as prophylaxis against ischemic events in patients with TIA, particularly when embolism is suspected.

The results of several randomized studies performed to date suggest but do not conclusively demonstrate a treatment benefit. Moreover, anticoagulation is associated with an increased risk of cerebral hemorrhage. Although the reported risks of hemorrhagic complications are probably lessened through control of hypertension and assiduous maintenance of the prothrombin time at 1.5 control values, the relatively low incidence of stroke 1 or more years after the onset of TIA (approximately 5% per year) provides little rationale for long-term anticoagulation. Furthermore, the incidence of stroke in patients with amaurosis fugax may be lower than that in patients with other types of TIA. Short-term anticoagulation may be of benefit when instituted in the first month or two following the onset of symptoms when the risk of stroke is thought to be greatest. It may be considered in patients who have noted a recent increase in the frequency of symptoms or in those whose symptoms persist or recur when they receive aspirin therapy.

Endarterectomy

Currently the third most commonly performed surgical procedure in the United States, carotid endarterectomy remains the subject of intense controversy. It has been employed to reduce the risk of future stroke in patients with asymptomatic bruits, carotid and vertebrobasilar TIA, and completed strokes. The only large, prospective, controlled study comparing endarterectomy with nonsurgical management showed that the incidence of stroke was lower in the surgical group following discharge from the hospital but that when perioperative morbidity and mortality were taken into consideration the results of medical and surgical therapy were comparable. Even assuming that surgical techniques have improved and that operative risk has diminished, as reported by several centers, the existing data are insufficient to identify which if any specific groups of patients stand to benefit from the procedure. Until more facts become available, surgical intervention should be restricted to those patients judged to have the highest risk of stroke and the lowest operative risk. The best results to date have been achieved in patients with amaurosis or hemispheric TIA who have demonstrable atherosclerotic disease of the extracranial internal carotid artery on the side appropriate to the symptoms. Given our present state of knowledge, carotid endarterectomy *should not* be performed for the following: (1) vertebrobasilar TIA including cases associated with binocular transient visual loss, (2) asymptomatic carotid bruit, (3) mild degrees of stenosis or ulceration in symptomatic patients, and (4) complete occlusion of the internal carotid artery or significant stenosis of the carotid siphon. In addition, patients over the age of 70 and those with significant cardiac or pulmonary disease represent poor surgical risks and, in general, should not undergo either angiography or endarterectomy. Several prospective randomized trials comparing modern endarterectomy techniques to medical management are currently underway and can be expected to clarify the merits of and the indications for this procedure.

Bibliography

1. Burde RM, Savino PJ, Trobe JD: "Transient visual loss," in *Clinical Decisions in Neuro-Ophthalmology*. St Louis, CV Mosby Co, 1985.
2. Caplan LR: Carotid-artery disease. *N Engl J Med* 1986; 315:886–888.
3. Grotta JC: Current medical and surgical therapy for cerebrovascular disease. *N Engl J Med* 1987; 317:1505–1508.
4. Sandok BA, Furlan AJ, Whisnant JP, et al: Guidelines for the management of transient ischemic attacks. *Mayo Clin Proc* 1978; 53:665–674.

Approach 2 _____

Peter J. Savino, M.D.

The patient is a 62-year-old woman with several episodes of blurred vision lasting "several minutes." In this age group several entities of neuro-ophthalmic importance come to mind. It would be critical to have more information about the patient's pattern of visual loss. For example, if she had cross-covered each eye and knew that the blurred vision was in one eye or the other, this would limit the diagnostic possibilities to the anterior visual pathways. If, however, the blurred vision was bilateral and simultaneous, this would more likely, although not necessarily, put the lesion more posteriorly. She might also be experiencing transient homonymous hemianopsia, which a patient will many times confuse with a loss of vision in the eye on the side of the homonymous defect.

If the patient could determine that the loss was in one eye while the other eye remained perfectly normal and there was no ocular cause for this, e.g., intermittent angle closure or bleeding from an anterior-chamber lens, several neuro-ophthalmic disorders should be investigated:

1. Giant cell arteritis is a possibility in this woman, and transient visual loss prior to ischemic optic neuropathy is not uncommon in these patients. Therefore a sedimentation rate determination is indicated and a thorough history as to the signs and symptoms of polymyalgia rheumatica, jaw claudication, weight loss, etc.

2. Amaurosis fugax on the basis of carotid artery disease can be ruled out with noninvasive testing. Duplex scanning is the state-of-the-art method that should be employed.

3. Cardiac lesions may cause unilateral visual loss. A good cardiac evaluation by a cardiologist should obviate the need for

more sophisticated testing such as echocardiography or Holter monitoring.

If the patient instead states that the visual loss is bilateral and simultaneous or if it is homonymous in nature, then the problem resides in the retrochiasmal, most likely occipital, area. Testing that should be conducted at this time includes the following:

1. Cardiac evaluation should be undertaken since the most likely cause for vertebrobasilar transient ischemia is cardiac arrhythmia or embolization to the vertebrobasilar system from a heart valve, intraventricular mass lesion such as a myxoma, or a clot overlying an area of ischemic myocardium.

2. A thorough history of migraine phenomena should be elicited since the most frequent cause of homonymous defects is migraine.

3. Visual fields should be performed to see whether there is a fixed deficit. If there is, a CT scan should be performed.

If the patient is unable to determine whether the visual loss is unilateral, bilateral, or homonymous, then all of the aforementioned testing should be done.

Changing Discs and Abnormal Fields—But the Patient Just Wants a Pair of Glasses!

APPROACH 1

Lanning B. Kline, M.D.

APPROACH 2

James Goodwin, M.D.

Case 19 _____

Changing Discs and Abnormal Fields—But the Patient Just Wants a Pair of Glasses!

A 57-year-old man returns for his biannual refraction with vague visual complaints both for near and distance. He is found to have 20/20 vision in each eye with a small change in refraction and reads 4 point at near with a +0.50-D increase in his add. The intraocular pressure is normal, but examination of his discs finds cup-to-disc ratios of 0.4 and 0.6 in the right and left eyes. The records show 0.2 for each eye several years before.

A computerized visual field is obtained and shows generalized depression in each eye with greater loss of sensitivity on the temporal side. A skull x-ray with special views of the sella are normal.

The patient requests his prescription for glasses. Is any further workup indicated?

Summary _____

This case is a clinical snakepit: what to do with an indifferent patient who has optic nerve signs of glaucoma, normal intraocular pressures, a visual field suggestive of a chiasmal tumor, and a normal skull x-ray?

Both of the discussants express the opinion that manual Goldmann perimetry is a more specific method of discriminating glaucoma from a chiasmal lesion in this patient. Dr. Kline stresses the importance of observing whether the field defect respects the horizontal or vertical midlines and whether it is connected to the blind spot or to fixation.

Dr. Goodwin reminds us that our patient can harbor a chiasmal mass (including an aneurysm) and still have normal skull x-ray findings. While not minimizing the usefulness of this simple test, a normal result should not deter the ophthalmologist from referring the patient for a computed tomography (CT) scan.

Both of the discussants believe that neuro-ophthalmologic lesions are better evaluated with manual perimetry than with an automated visual field testing device. It is important to be aware that the experts evaluate the fields of these patients by using manual perimetry.

257

Approach 1 —————————————————

Lanning B. Kline, M.D.

The clinical findings in this 57-year-old man include (1) 20/20 vision in both eyes; (2) "normal" intraocular pressure; (3) asymmetrical optic disc cupping; (4) bilateral visual field "depression," with greatest loss temporally; and (5) normal skull films.

The differential diagnosis lies between "normal-tension" glaucoma and nonglaucomatous disc excavation due to some other form of optic nerve disease (e.g., compressive, inflammatory, ischemic).

To begin with, further office testing is essential prior to considering additional workup. Assessment of color vision with Ishihara pseudoisochromatic color plates is a valuable measure of optic nerve function. Pupillary reactions should also be recorded, with careful testing for a relative afferent defect (Gunn pupil). Examination plates are available to measure contrast sensitivity, also useful in detecting optic nerve disease. In general, all these parameters of optic nerve function are disturbed much earlier in the course of a nonglaucomatous optic neuropathy than in glaucoma.

Careful examination of the optic discs may provide additional clues as to the presence or absence of glaucoma. In a study of nonglaucomatous disc cupping, Trobe et al.[1] found two ophthalmoscopic findings to be of diagnostic help: (1) pallor of the neuroretinal rim suggested nonglaucomatous atrophy, and (2) focal or diffuse obliteration of the rim was more common in glaucoma. Therefore, the status of the remaining neuroretinal tissue in our patient's optic discs needs careful observation.

As a general rule optic disc cupping and visual field defects occur early in glaucoma.[2] Acuity is usually spared until field loss is extensive. In contrast, decreased visual acuity is an early sign of compressive optic neuropathy, as is field loss. Optic disc changes (cupping, pallor) occur later in the clinical course.[3] The progressive changes in our patient's optic discs with good Snellen acuity is thus more suggestive of glaucomatous disc damage.

Of greatest importance in determining further patient evaluation is the visual field examination. An automated study demonstrated "generalized depression," with the major loss temporally in each eye. The critical question in terms of field testing is whether the defects have respect for the horizontal or vertical meridian and what is this relationship to the blind spot (Fig 19–1). If the field defects do respect the vertical meridian, then the patient has a bitemporal hemianopia, and workup for chiasmal disease is indicated. However, bilateral superior nerve fiber bundle defects indicate bilateral optic nerve disease and the likelihood of normal-tension glaucoma. In this situation, medication to lower the intraocular pressure is indicated.

I would favor careful visual field examination prior to further workup for intracranial disease. My bias would be to repeat the visual fields examination on a bowl perimeter. If a bitemporal field defect with respect for the vertical meridian is present, then neuroradiological evaluation is needed. Skull films with special views of the sella were ordered. This study assesses bone changes but provides no soft-tissue detail. Cranial CT should be the initial study obtained. The clinician must communicate his concerns to the radiologist and emphasize the need for careful study of the anterior visual pathways. Merely asking the radiologist to "rule out brain tumor" is insufficient and may lead to an inadequate examination and a false-negative study.

CT evaluation of the optic chiasm requires proper attention to technique, including multiple projections (axial, coronal), thin-section tomography (≤ 5 mm), and intravenous contrast medium. Criteria for detecting chiasmal disease with CT have been reported.[4]

Magnetic resonance imaging (MRI) could be performed instead of CT. Advantages of MRI include the absence of ionizing radiation and no need for intravenous contrast. However, bone changes are not detectable with this technique. MRI is still in a relatively early stage of development. Future improvements in spatial and contrast

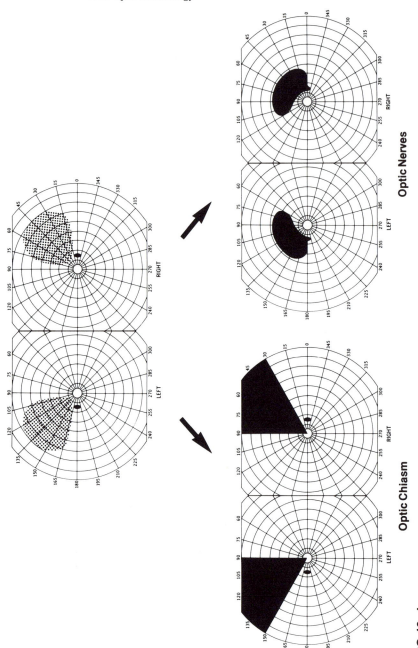

FIG 19–1.
The critical question in a patient with bitemporal field loss: does the defect go to fixation (chiasmatic lesion) or to the blind spot with or without respect for the horizontal meridian (optic nerve lesion)?

resolution will probably eventually make MRI the procedure of choice in chiasmal evaluation.

In summary, I would initially perform additional office tests on the patient to measure optic nerve function including color vision, pupillary examination, and contrast sensitivity. Next, visual fields need to be re-examined, probably with a bowl perimeter, to see whether or not a bitemporal hemianopia is present. If an intracranial lesion is suspected, cranial CT or MRI should be performed and the radiologist told of the precise area requiring study.

References

1. Trobe JD, Glaser JS, Cassady J, et al: Nonglaucomatous excavation of the optic disc. *Arch Ophthalmol* 1980; 98:1046–1050.
2. Kolker AE, Hetherington J: Becker-Shaffer's Diagnosis and Therapy of the Glaucomas, ed 5. St Louis, CV Mosby Co, 1983, pp 170.
3. Kuppersmith MJ, Krohn D: Cupping of the optic disc and compressive lesions of the anterior visual pathways. *Ann Ophthalmol* 1984; 16:948–953.
4. Kline LB, Vitek JJ, Acker JD: Computed tomography in the evaluation of the optic chiasm. *Surv Ophthalmol* 1983; 27:387–396.

Approach 2 _____

James Goodwin, M.D.

A 57-year-old man comes to his ophthalmologist with vague visual complaints, and examination reveals larger physiological cups than were described several years previously. Visual acuity was normal, but there was generalized loss of visual field sensitivity in each eye, and the loss was greater in the temporal field than in the nasal. The sella turcica is normal on plain skull x-rays.

Is Further Workup Indicated? Yes

Patients with visual disorders that affect primarily the extra-foveal visual field, even though the "central field" is involved, often offer little or no complaint, and the physician cannot rely upon them to push for workup. Most ophthalmologists would not hesitate to push further if the patient were vociferous about his failing vision or if the Snellen acuity were reduced without adequate explanation. On the other hand, a satisfied patient with 20/20 acuity may slip through the system unnoticed and yet be harboring a serious progressive disease. Prior to the advent of office computerized perimeters, the visual field examination was not a major part of the routine office visit. It is natural that in the course of patient care one looks less and less for the things that one sees least. Thus when faced with an uncommon disorder, the unwary ophthalmologist no longer utilizes the tools with which to look for the disorder, and it is missed.

Patients with 20/20 vision and visual complaints are not common, and there is a tendency to regard them as neurotic. Many physicians do not acknowledge that a loss of the extrafoveal visual field produces symptoms—in fact, however, these patients do not see as well as they did before, and they may complain of it. Since the central resolving power is still good, they read the Snellen chart with ease, and the quality of the visual experience is something other than simple blurring. This leads to the "vague" quality of the symptoms.

History

The first aspect of additional workup is more detailed history taking. This utilizes the most expensive and scarce resource of the medical complex—the physician's time. Nonetheless, neurological diagnosis is based more solidly on history than on physical examination, and a few minutes taken to pin down the exact details will often save a lot of unnecessary lab work. The patient should be asked whether his visual disturbance is generalized or localized within the visual fields. Much can be brought out by asking him to describe the activity he was performing when he first noticed the problem. What was he looking at then, and what type of viewing—dim or bright environment, light or dark colors— makes the visual defect most pronounced? This type of questioning often induces patients to recall experiences that indicate a localized field defect.

Has the patient tried covering each eye to determine whether the problem is monocular or binocular? If the symptom is ongoing at the time of the examination, the patient should be asked to cover each eye and to describe what he sees. Is the examiner's face symmetrical in color and clarity? Are straight edges in the room still straight? This is a sort of environmental Amsler grid test.

The history is also important to establish the time course of the problem. Slowly progressive symptoms with normal ocular examination findings should indicate tumor compression of the anterior visual pathways (optic nerves, chiasm, optic tract) as the principal diagnosis. Remember, *chronic optic neuritis* does not occur often enough to make this a smart diagnosis in the setting of slowly progressive visual loss or symptoms of the same.

Visual Fields

The next element in further workup is further visual field assessment. Notice, the patient has not even left the physician's office yet. I have developed a strong bias toward Goldmann perimetry as a *neurodiagnostic field examination*. The arrays of numbers delivered by the threshold programs of computerized perimeters may give some vague impression of the morphology of field defects, but the quality of this aspect is severely wanting. Goldmann dynamic perimetry may not give as complete a depiction of threshold at all points in the field and may or may not be as good for quantitative followup, but it is a time honored way of discovering field patterns that have exquisite localizing value. I do not expect the busy ophthalmologist to spend his own time doing manual perimetry, but a technician can be trained to perform sensitive and reproducible examinations, and the physician should be prepared to check critical areas of the field. This is not very time-consuming—honest. Still, you may prefer to refer this type of patient to your neuro-ophthalmologist; his children need new shoes anyway.

The computer field in this case indicates generalized loss of sensitivity, and this translates into concentric contraction of isopters in the dynamic field. Greater loss on the temporal side is the warning flag since glaucoma reliably produces greater loss in the nasal fields. The earliest and most pronounced field defect in glaucoma is in the arcuate or Bjerrum region, which starts out as a narrow zone at the blind spot and expands into a broad area nasal to the fixation point. Even if the patient has glaucomatous atrophy of the nerve heads (enlarging physiological cups), the described field loss is probably from another disease!

Bitemporal field defects are the hallmark of disease, usually compression, at the optic chiasm. The axons coming from ganglion cells nasal to the fovea all cross in the chiasm, so they are relatively tethered and unable to accommodate compressive forces from below, or so the story goes. Regardless of the neuromythology we use to explain it, the fact remains that most patients with compression of the chiasm have bitemporal field defects and most patients with glaucoma have Bjerrum area nasal defects. After all, there is nothing about glaucoma that prevents lesions at the chiasm and vice versa.

Optic Disc Morphology

Joel Glaser recently discussed whether acute anterior ischemic optic neuropathy (AION) occurs preferentially in small crowded discs having small physiological cups: this is a proposal that is going around. He and several colleagues expert in optic disc observation estimated physiological cup ratios in a large number of nerve heads in stereo fundus photographs. He found that the interobserver agreement for this measurement was dismally poor. Thus, if our patient's previous cup determination was done by another ophthalmologist, it is far from clear that the change from 0.2 cups to 0.5 is a reliable indicator of change. This man may not have glaucoma at all.

Neuroimaging

The final aspect of the diagnostic process in this case is identification of the problem that is probably going on at the optic chiasm. The most common lesion to produce bitemporal field defects is the pituitary adenoma, which is endocrinologically silent in the majority of men who, therefore, present only after compression of the optic chiasm produces visual symptoms. The sella is almost always enlarged by symptomatic pituitary adenomas, so this would not be the first diagnosis in this patient.

Cushing's syndrome of the optic chiasm refers to patients who present with progressive bitemporal field loss and a normal sella on plain x-ray studies. Harvey Cushing indicated that the differential diagnosis in these cases includes (1) craniopharyngioma, (2) tuberculum sella meningioma, and (3) aneurysm. All of these lesions may cause visual symptoms with normal skull x-ray findings. Thus, screening for chiasmal compressive lesions cannot be done adequately by plain skull x-rays or even tomograms since the bones of the sella region may be normal. CT with thin cuts through the suprasellar cistern or MRI is needed. Aneurysms still require cerebral angiography to be excluded, though the large suprasellar aneurysms can be distinguished on high-quality CT with infusion and on MRI. Newer pulse sequences in MRI can distinguish flowing blood from calcification, both of which produce black "signal void" areas on routine T_1 and T_2 weighted studies. This is a problem area since a large aneurysm may undergo thrombosis and become calcified, in which case it might be mistaken for a meningioma.

Conclusion

I see several cases a year in which the patient has been complaining about declining vision for years and either vision is normal or declining Snellen acuity has been documented but no diagnosis made. These patients have usually seen more than one ophthalmologist by the time they get to me. The diagnosis of chiasm or optic nerve compression is usually obvious when adequate visual field examination is done. It is mandatory that every ophthalmologist keep this kind of presentation in mind on a day-to-day basis and that adequate visual field examination be carried out on any patient who presents with unexplained visual loss or with visual symptoms that are not explained by the examination.

SECTION VII

Contact Lens and Refraction

Contact Lens Intolerance— Rather Fight or Switch?

APPROACH 1

David J. Fuerst, M.D.

APPROACH 2

Timothy T. McMahon, O.D., F.A.A.O.

Case 20 _____

Contact Lens Intolerance—Rather Fight or Switch?

A 24-year-old professional model complains of irritation in both eyes and an inability to tolerate her contact lenses for more than a few hours at a time. She has worn extended-wear soft contact lenses for 3 years without difficulty but lately has been wearing them as daily wear lenses.

Examination reveals 20/20 vision in each eye with a −7.00 D sphere. The conjunctivae are mildly injected, and there is a carpet of moderate-sized papillae superiorly in each eye.

The patient would like to continue wearing contact lenses, if possible. What is the best approach to this problem?

Summary

Almost all of us, regardless of subspecialization, have patients in our practices who wear contact lenses. Even those who do not fit lenses will occasionally be asked to "take a look." The case described here is common in that the patient has worn lenses for several years, is now just beginning to experience problems, and insists on wearing the lenses.

One of the two most common causes of contact lens intolerance is contact lens keratoconjunctivitis (CLK). The findings and treatment of this condition are described by Dr. Fuerst in his discussion. This condition appears to be an allergic reaction to the preservatives in contact lens solutions.

Dr. McMahon discusses the role of giant papillary conjunctivitis in contact lens intolerance. His approach is based on evaluating the severity of the disease and then customizing therapy depending on that evaluation.

Both of the discussions stress the importance of ruling out the less common conditions in the differential diagnosis prior to starting therapy. Most of the other disease processes will not respond to therapy that is intended as treatment for CLK or giant papillary conjunctivitis (GPC).

Approach 1

David J. Fuerst, M.D.

We are presented with a young woman who has successfully worn soft contact lenses for 3 years but now has had to change from extended-wear to daily-wear. She retains good visual acuity but has findings of conjunctival hyperemia and moderate-sized papillae superiorly.

Whenever a patient presents with contact lens intolerance, it is important to obtain a complete history including current symptoms and lens care regimen. Questions regarding the age of the current lenses, the frequency of obtaining new lenses, the use of lens care products (including saline solutions, surfactant-type cleaners, and enzyme), and the use of topical ophthalmic medications will help in diagnosing the probable etiology of the symptoms and therefore aid in choosing changes in the regimen to effect therapy. The patient should also be asked specifically about symptoms of itching, mucus production, awareness of the lens on the eye, excessive lens movement, or visual blurring.

A careful, systematic examination should include evaluation of the soft contact lens both on and off the eye. Lens discoloration and surface changes, warpage, nicks, and tears are evidence of lens aging. Deposits, especially protein, are most easily seen by gently drying the lens and observing it with the biomicroscope. Slit-lamp evaluation of the anterior segment should include examination of the eyelids, tear film, both the bulbar and tarsal conjunctivae, and cornea.

Particular attention should be paid to the location and character of papillae. This is done by eversion of the upper eyelid and examination with the biomicroscope using white light. Fluorescein may be instilled and a cobalt blue light used to highlight smaller papillae. Apical staining of macropapillae or giant papillae may be seen in more advanced cases. Occasionally, red-free light aids in the evaluation of the vascular pattern of the papillae. A baseline diagram or photograph of the papillae on the tarsal conjunctiva will help in monitoring the condition as well as the response to therapy.

Enlarged papillae are seen in many external eye diseases including superior limbic keratoconjunctivitis, vernal conjunctivitis, keratoconjunctivitis sicca, medicamentosa, staphylococcal blepharoconjunctivitis, allergic conjunctivitis, bacterial conjunctivitis, adenoviral infections, trachoma, inclusion conjunctivitis, and others. Any of these conditions may occur in a contact lens wearer. Once these entities are ruled out by the history and findings, CLK and GPC should be considered.

Contact Lens Keratoconjunctivitis

A mild, uniform papillary reaction of the superior tarsal conjunctiva is seen with CLK,[1] a condition with more severe involvement of the bulbar conjunctiva and cornea. Patients with CLK complain of lens intolerance, redness, burning, foreign body sensation, photophobia, and blurred vision. The keratoconjunctivopathy has a predilection for the superior aspects of the globe, an area that is partially covered by the upper eyelid. This condition, also described as a superior limbic keratoconjunctivitis–like problem in contact lens wearers (CL-SLK) is likely caused by preservatives, especially thimerosal, although ethylenediamine tetraacetic acid (EDTA), chlorhexidine, and other preservatives may be involved. Allergy to thimerosal, which is a type IV cell-mediated reaction, seems to require multiple exposures to this preservative over a prolonged time period. CLK occurs from 1 to 8 years after starting soft contact lens wear. CLK is much more common in daily-wear contact lens patients, probably because their lenses are in daily contact with the preservatives contained in many lens care products.

CLK must be treated initially by discontinuation of lens wear. Corneal findings may take weeks or months to resolve and may worsen considerably if any preservative-laden contact lens or other preservative-containing product is used. Many patients unfortunately continue at least occasional contact lens wear since they find that the visual blurring from the epithelial keratitis is improved with the contact lens on. Therapy with preservative-free artificial tears or a more viscous preparation such as unpreserved gum cellulose, 0.625%, is used. Steroid therapy is minimally helpful, if at all. Once all signs and symptoms resolve, a new soft contact lens may be used with a preservative-free cleaning program including heat or hydrogen peroxide disinfection. Mechanical surface cleaning with baby shampoo and unpreserved saline is an alternative to using commercial contact lens cleaning solutions. If a product containing any preservatives is used on the lens, multiple rinses with unpreserved saline should be performed prior to inserting the lens. Aerosolized saline is preferred. Alternatively, a rigid gas-permeable contact lens may be tried, with unpreserved saline rinses before lens insertion.

Giant Papillary Conjunctivitis

The other important contact lens–related syndrome with a papillary conjunctivitis is GPC.[2] This condition is characterized by symptoms of morning mucus production variably decreased vision, mild itching, and an awareness of the lens during wear. This condition usually presents within a few months of starting lens wear. Signs include macropapillae (0.3 to 1.0 mm) or giant papillae (over 1.0 mm) with thickened tarsal conjunctiva, mucus in the conjunctival cul-de-sac, and hyperemia. In hydrogel lens wearers, the papillae are most prominent near the tarsal fold, with the least involvement nearest the eyelid margin. Examination of the contact lens will demonstrate surface deposits usually appearing as an irregular filmy coating.

The pathogenesis of GPC is thought to be a combination of mechanical and immunologic factors. The contact lens causes chronic irritation of the conjunctiva while presenting foreign antigens to this surface. These antigens may include bacteria, foreign proteins, or mucoproteins from the patient that are antigenically altered by the chemicals or heat used for contact lens sterilization. Type I (IgE) and type IV (cutaneous basophil) hypersensitivity reactions are thought to play a role, with eosinophils, basophils, and mast cells variably noted in conjunctival epithelium.

Treatment of GPC may be accomplished by cessation of lens wear, adapting a meticulous and frequent lens cleaning regimen, changing to a different hydrogel lens, or switching to a nonhydrogel lens. Since most soft lens wearers are highly motivated to continue lens wear, an attempt at continuing lens wear with a modified cleaning schedule is almost always considered. Unless the signs and symptoms are mild, discontinuing lens wear for several days or weeks is recommended. Depending on the severity of symptoms, treatment with cromolyn sodium and/or steroids may be started. When the conjunctival hyperemia has substantially subsided (papillae may still be present), new lenses are dispensed; although any lens may be associated with GPC, I find that glyceryl-methyl methacrylate (CMI) daily-wear lenses are best tolerated. A new cleaning regimen is carefully outlined, including daily cleaning with a commercial surfactant, hydrogen peroxide sterilization, and frequent enzyme treatments. If signs and symptoms recur, consider using cromolyn sodium topically, four times per day, and continuing lens wear. If contact lens intolerance is still noted despite the combination of a new lens, conscientious cleaning regimen, and topical cromolyn, a recommendation is made to change to a rigid gas-permeable lens or abandon contact lens wear completely.

New Products

New contact lens products have been developed that will benefit individuals with CLK or GPC. Preservatives such as polyaminopropyl biguanide (Dymed) and Polyquaternium-1 (Polyquad) have recently become available and may be used instead of thimerosal in solutions and surfactant-type cleaners. Less than 20% of soft contact lens care products contain thimerosal, as listed in the 1988 *Physicians' Desk Reference* for Ophthalmology, and several brands of unpreserved saline are now available. Hydrogen peroxide sterilization was recently introduced and can be used with any currently marketed contact lens. This is a simple, effective means of sterilization that does not leave preservatives on the lens. A new enzyme product, subtilisin (Ultrazyme), can be used simultaneously with hydrogen peroxide sterilization, which makes this important step in contact lens cleaning easier and therefore encourages compliance. Development of the disposable extended-wear contact lens may obviate the need for using any preservatives. Frequent replacement of this lens will also limit the amount of protein deposition, thereby decreasing or eliminating the need for enzyme.

Other considerations for the contact lens–intolerant patient include spectacle correction and refractive surgery. Refractive surgery should only be contemplated if the anterior segment is free of inflammation and any secondary corneal changes are stable. Caution must be exercised since subtle surface changes of the cornea may lead to epithelial problems after refractive surgery with resultant complications.

In summary, the two most common causes of contact lens–associated papillary conjunctivitis are CLK and GPC. A history, including detailed questions regarding the lens care regimen and symptoms, combined with a biomicroscopic examination will usually disclose the etiology. Discontinuing contact lens wear until the conjunctival (or corneal) signs and symptoms abate is almost always necessary. For CLK, contact lens wear may be resumed if a preservative-free lens care regimen is used. For GPC, a strict contact lens cleaning program including the use of enzyme will often allow successful resumption of contact lens wear.

References

1. Wilson FM II: Preservative-induced contact-lens keratoconjunctivitis. Presented at the Francis I. Proctor Foundation 40th Anniversary Symposium, San Francisco, Sept. 14, 1987.
2. Greiner JV, Fowler SA, Allansmith MR: Giant papillary conjunctivitis, in Dabezies OH (ed): *Contact Lenses, the CLAO Guide to Basic Science and Clinical Practice*, Orlando, Fla, Grune & Stratton, 1984.

Approach 2

Timothy T. McMahon, O.D., F.A.A.O.

The history for this patient is consistent with the diagnosis of GPC, a condition associated with contact lens wear. The management of this problem depends upon an accurate diagnosis and selection of a suitable treatment regimen. It seems appropriate to begin with the symptoms and physical findings of GPC, followed by the differential diagnosis and the treatment options, in order to explain the specific management rationale for this patient.

Physical Findings and Symptoms

GPC has been identified in patients with corneal and scleral surface foreign bodies, including contact lenses, corneal and scleral sutures, ocular prostheses, and extruded scleral buckles. The incidence of GPC is estimated to be between 1% and 10% in hard-lens wearers and 10% and 15% in soft-lens wearers.[1, 2] Presenting symptoms include itching, burning, blurred vision, mucus discharge, photosensitivity, conjunctival hyperemia, and ptosis with eyelid thickening. Contact lens wearers will additionally report heavy lens deposits, decreased lens tolerance, and excessive lens movement.

On examination of contact lens wearers, visual acuity with contact lenses may be reduced to 20/200. This is due to lens deposits, tearing from photosensitivity, or rarely, an irregular corneal surface. Spectacle-corrected vision is only rarely reduced. The eyelids may appear diffusely thickened. Mucus is commonly found in the canthal regions, particularly nasally. On upper-lid eversion, the tarsal conjunctiva may present with a variety of findings including hyperemia, follicles, papillae, mucus strands, and patchy fibrosis of the conjunctival substantia propria. Allansmith et al.[3] and Greiner et al.[1] have described four stages of GPC that are based primarily upon the clinical appearance of the superior tarsal conjunctiva. In stage 1 the patient experiences mild itching after lens removal and can find mucus in the nasal canthus upon awakening in the morning. No physical findings are seen on slit-lamp examination. Stage 1 symptoms are rarely elicited. Usually, the syndrome is not recognized by the patient or doctor until at least stage 2. In stage 2, itching and mucus discharge are more notable, and contact lens coating becomes evident. Small- to moderate-sized papillae and occasionally a few giant papillae are found on the superior tarsal conjunctiva. The conjunctiva appears mildly hyperemic and edematous. For stage 3 the itching, mucus discharge, and lens coating become more severe. Excessive lens movement is noted as well as decreased tolerance. Giant papillae are always found at this stage, and mild lid edema is usually present. In stage 4 disease, there is a total loss of contact lens tolerance, giant papillae are florid, ptosis is present because of lid thickening, mucus secretions are heavy, and a foreign body sensation with and without the lenses in place is common.

Involvement of the cornea is rare in GPC. When there is corneal involvement, scattered or confluent punctate epitheliopathy is found, and the surface may be mildly irregular. In my experience, corneal involvement has been present only in extremely acute cases when there are heavy deposits on the contact lenses. The lens deposits probably act mechanically to disturb the corneal surface. The inferior tarsal conjunctiva may have follicles (common) and papillae (uncommon) and may be hyperemic. Limbal chemosis is rare and mild. Mild diffuse bulbar conjunctival hyperemia is common.

The onset of symptoms is gradual, over a period of days to weeks. In contact lens wearers the initial reported symptom is usually an increase in contact lens deposits. Mild irritation and/or itching follows during lens wear. If lens use continues, wearing time begins to shorten because of discomfort. It is common for patients, at this point, to think that the problem is a "spoiled" or "old" lens and to seek a replacement pair of lenses. New lenses are generally palliative for several days to weeks and occasionally for periods longer than a month. When symptoms reappear, then they come into the office for examination. In individuals who persist with lens wear, excessive lens coating, lid swelling, and irritation as well as ptosis with and without a lens in place, may occur. In extreme cases limbal and corneal changes may also appear.

Histopathology and Pathogenesis

The histopathologic findings of the affected conjunctiva include mast cells, found primarily in the epithelium, as well as plasma cells and eosinophils, principally located in the substantia propria.[3, 4] Of significance is the presence of basophils in the epithelium and substantia propria, which indicates a type of delayed hypersensitivity immunologic response.[3, 5] Immunoglobulin levels (IgE, IgG, and IgM) are also elevated and/or present in the tears.[6, 7] This constellation of immunologic responses suggest a combined type I IgE-mediated hypersensitivity and a type IV delayed hypersensitivity.

Available evidence and theory regarding the pathogenesis of GPC center around mechanical trauma from the contact lens to the tarsal conjunctiva and immunologic response to lens surface antigens, presumed to be deposits accumulated on the contact lens. Greiner et al.[1] theorize that mechanical trauma from the lens rubbing against the tarsal conjunctiva damages the epithelial surface and results in the degranulation of mast cells, which causes tissue edema (and itching) and exposure to antigens that would not normally penetrate intact conjunctival epithelium. Exposure to these antigens would then generate a release of inflammatory mediators in the substantia propria followed by the influx of inflammatory cells. One could also postulate that a delayed hypersensitivity process initially generates the response after a sensitizing dose of antigen. Mechanical trauma may then enhance the response by damaging the edematous conjunctival epithelium and exposing more and potentially different antigens for response. The major factors of clinical importance are that both lens-induced trauma and an immunologic response are involved. To resolve and prevent the disease, both factors must be taken into consideration.

Differential Diagnosis

1. Vernal keratoconjunctivitis (VKC)
2. Superior limbic keratoconjunctivitis associated with contact lens wear (CL-SLK)
3. Atopic keratoconjunctivitis
4. Allergic conjunctivitis
5. Viral conjunctivitis
6. Chlamydial conjunctivitis
7. Bacterial conjunctivitis

The differential diagnosis of GPC represents those disorders in which papillae have been found as a distinctive feature. A papillary response by the tarsal conjunctiva is not unique to GPC. However, the historical information in conjunction with the physical findings makes the diagnosis relatively straightforward.

The features differentiating VKC from GPC include predominance in males, an atopic history, and an age of onset commonly before 10 years, which is usually earlier than initial contact lens wear. Recurrences of VKC, in most cases, are more seasonal than with GPC. Corneal and limbal involvement are prominent features when found, and itching is more profound in VKC. In my experience, patients with inactive or active VKC do not tolerate contact lenses from the start. Signs and symptoms of VKC occur without the presence of a foreign body such as a contact lens. There is always a foreign body involved in GPC.

CL-SLK may present with papillary hypertrophy; however, this is not an impressive feature of the disorder. The bulbar conjunctival and corneal changes are more prominent and can be utilized to differentiate the two diseases. Contact lens deposits are common in CL-SLK, but itching is not found.

Atopic keratoconjunctivitis presents with papillary hypertrophy as a prominent feature. It may be differentiated from GPC by the presence of systemic findings such as atopic dermatitis, asthma, hay fever, and rhinitis. The ocular findings in addition to superior and inferior tarsal papillae include scaly, wrinkled, swollen, and inflamed skin of the eyelids, corneal vascularization, and cataracts. The findings are always bilateral. Itching and photophobia are common features. Eosinophils are a prominent feature of conjunctival scrapings, but mast cells are not as abundant as in GPC. These findings are present with and without contact lens wear.

Allergic dermatoconjunctivitis (contact allergy) can be confused with GPC. The itching, mild chemosis, marked conjunctival hyperemia, eosinophilia and mild papillary response are similar to GPC. The eczematous dermatitis tends to be the prominent feature, however. Ocular medications and cosmetics are common causes. The prominent eyelid features, rhinitis, and continuation of symptoms following lens removal serve to differentiate the two.

In viral and chlamydial disease a heavy follicular response may be misdiagnosed as GPC. However, the follicular response is generally greater for the inferior palpebral conjunctival surface than the superior surface, and giant papillae are not found. Adenopathy of the preauricular lymph nodes is a common feature of viral disease but is not found in GPC. The symptoms also tend to persist for extended periods after the lens is removed, which is contrary to the natural history of GPC.

Bacterial infections are usually easily differentiated by the purulent discharge, conjunctival hyperemia, and hemorrhages. Papillary hypertrophy and giant papillae are secondary features.

Treatment Options

The management of GPC associated with contact lens wear can be divided into three phases: (1) treating the active disease, (2) returning the patient to contact lens wear, and (3) preventing recurrences.

When a patient presents with symptomatic GPC, the initial treatment regimen found in Table 20–1 is recommended. I recommend steroid use only in severe acute presentations.

TABLE 20–1.

Treatment of Symptomatic Contact Lens–induced GPC*

Symptom	Treatment
Severe (uncommon)	
Pain or marked discomfort	Discontinue contact lens use
Decreased vision	Topical steroids qid for 4 days[8]
Marked ptosis	Cromolyn sodium 4% qid for 4 weeks
Moderate mucus discharge	Cold compresses bid
Heavy lens deposits	
Moderate photosensitivity	
Moderate (common)	
Itching or discomfort	Discontinue contact lens use
Ptosis	Cromolyn sodium qid for 2–4 weeks
Mucus discharge	Cold compresses bid
Moderate to heavy lens deposits	
Mild photosensitivity	
Mild (common)	
Itching or discomfort	Discontinue contact lens use
Mild mucus discharge	Cold compresses bid
Moderate to heavy lens deposits	
Mild photosensitivity	
Minimal (common)	
Mild to moderate lens deposits	Discontinue contact lens use

*Table represents symptoms of GPC without contact lenses on the eye; qid, four times daily; bid, twice daily.

What constitutes the resolution of active GPC is not well defined clinically. Symptoms always resolve before the signs. With removal of the source of the inflammatory response (i.e., the contact lens), the disease is self-limited. In moderate to severe cases the treatment is directed primarily at bringing symptomatic relief and secondarily at aiding resolution of signs. I consider the disease resolved when all of the following occur: the patient is asymptomatic; the *apices* of the papillae no longer stain; all papillae are smaller than 1 mm in diameter; the tarsal conjunctiva is no longer hyperemic; and all corneal, limbal, and ptotic changes return to normal. The papillary and substantia propria conjunctival changes may take months or years to disappear. Prohibiting patients from using contact lenses during this period is unnecessarily conservative.

The return to contact lens wear of patient with GPC requires special consideration. Refitting should focus on providing a lens that is tolerated by the patient and that limits the mechanical irritation to the tarsal conjunctiva and a lens care regimen that is the least irritating/sensitizing yet most effective possible. It is very common for patients not to be comfortable wearing contact lenses after GPC (whether or not there has been a long hiatus from lens wear). Soft lenses generally are the most comfortable material available today; however, the incidence of GPC appears to be greater for soft lenses than for the other types of contact lenses. Additionally, the diameters of soft lenses are quite large compared with their rigid-lens counterparts. Therefore, to reduce mechanical insult, limit immunologic response, and provide a physically tolerable lens tends to require compromise. Ideally one would want a material that can be fit with very small diameters, be very wettable and resistant to deposits, be comfortable, afford good vision, and be physiologically well tolerated by the cornea. Of the currently available materials polymethylmethacrylate (PMMA) fills more of these requirements than the others. However, in the patient with GPC, after active disease tolerance to rigid materials is generally poor, especially in prior wearers of soft lenses. Therefore, I often have found it necessary to refit patients with soft lens materials. Ultimately the choice of material is most strongly based on patient comfort.

If a soft-lens material is selected, a low–water content lens is recommended because of its greater resistance to deposits. I have not seen a benefit or detriment in switching brands of lenses of similar water content and lens class. Clinical experience suggests that it may be beneficial to avoid lenses in Food and Drug Administration (FDA) groups II and IV (greater than 1% mole fraction of methacrylic acid). Those types in groups II and IV whose surface has been treated to alter surface electrical charges may act like those lenses in groups I and III (less than 1% mole fraction of methacrylic acid). The FDA has recently developed a new method of classifying soft hydrogel lens polymers on the basis of water content and the fraction of methacrylic acid in the material. Methacrylic acid is useful in elevating water content but also presents potential reactivity problems with solutions and molecules because the lens surface tends to have patches of polar groups exposed to the environment that allow other charged groups to bind to them. There is some belief that tear deposits, particularly proteins, bind at these sights. Because tear proteins may act as antigens in the GPC pathological process it may be wise to avoid lenses suspected of a greater affinity for proteins.[9] These comments are based on anecdotal cases reported to me and my own clinical experience. Definitive studies in this area are lacking.

Limiting the size of the lens, in theory, reduces the surface area of the lens in contact with the tarsal conjunctiva, thus reducing the mechanical insult upon this tissue. For rigid lens materials this is relatively easy. Rigid lenses should be refitted by using an intrapalpebral method, positioning the lens so that it is not under either lid in open primary gaze, and using lens diameters between 7.5 and 8.5 mm where possible. Also, edge design appears to be critically important. Keeping the edge lift and thickness to a minimum is helpful. It is less practical to fit small, soft-lens materials than standard sizes (14.0 to 14.8 mm), but Bausch & Lomb, American Hydron, Aquaflex (Cooper Co), Sola-Syntex, and several custom laboratories can provide small, low-water materials. A diameter between 12.5 and 13.8 mm is recommended to afford reasonable stability and tolerable corneal coverage. In the order of frequency, my selection of materials has been (1) small-diameter, low–water content hydrogels; (2) small-diameter PMMA lenses; and (3) small-diameter, siloxane/acrylate gas-permeable lenses. Future use of fluorocarbon designs or fluorinated siloxane/acrylate lenses may be beneficial due to the deposit resistance of these materials.

Because there is evidence of an immunologic response in GPC and some belief that proteinaceous deposits may be a stimulating factor, the cleaning of contact lenses should be emphasized to patients following the return to contact lens wear. Encourage patient compliance in frequent and vigorous use of surfactants and enzymatic cleaners. I recommend preservative-free products where possible in that preservatives, although it has not been proved, potentially play a role in this syndrome. The use of rehydrating or rewetting drops will help reduce mechanical irritation to the conjunctival surface. This philosophy exists for both rigid and soft lenses.

The wearing schedule should be limited to daily wear. Recurrences almost always occur if extended wear is begun or restarted. As a precaution I generally place patients on a limited wearing schedule of 8 to 10 hours per day or less, to be gradually reached over a period of a week.

For the patient described in this case history the salient features are occupation (high cosmetic motivation), high myopia, decreasing wearing time, papillary response, and prior extended wear of soft lenses. Initially, this patient would be removed from wearing lenses until the apical staining of the papillae, mucus discharge, etc., resolved. Should this patient wish to return to lenses, I would initially recommend a small-diameter, low–water content hydrogel lens; a limited wearing schedule; use of unpreserved cleaners and saline; daily thermal or peroxide disinfection; and twice-weekly enzymatic cleaning. If the patient proved to be intolerant to this type of lens, 4% cromolyn sodium twice a day (before and after lens wear) would be recommended for 2 to 4 weeks. After this period cromolyn would be recommended on a symptomatic basis. If soft lenses continue to be poorly tolerated, an office trial of PMMA lenses would be attempted and ordered if tolerable. In my experience, this is only rarely useful in prior soft-lens wearers. Additional problems to rule out that may add to or be responsible for contact lens intolerance in this case would be tear insufficiency, blepharitis, meibomian gland dysfunction, and excessive makeup in the tear film. At times these underlying problems have been more a cause of patients' symptoms than mild GPC. Should all efforts fail, discontinuing contact lens wear would be advised for 6 to 8 months, and glasses would be prescribed. Rigid or hydrogel materials could be tried again at that time. If tolerance to contact lenses is still poor, then the use of spectacles or refractive surgery would be advised.

References

1. Greiner JV, Fowler SA, Allansmith MR: Giant papillary conjunctivitis in contact lenses, in Dabezies OH (ed): *The CLAO Guide to Basic Science and Clinical Practice,* vol 2. Orlando, Fla, Grune & Stratton, 1984, pp 1–15.
2. Korb DR, Allansmith MR, Greiner JV, et al: Prevalance of conjunctival changes in wearers of hard contact lenses. *Am J Ophthalmol* 1980; 90:336.
3. Allansmith MR, Korb DR, Griner JV, et al: Giant papillary conjunctivitis in contact lens wearers. *Am J Ophthalmol* 1977; 83:697.
4. Allansmith MR, Korb DR, Greiner JV: Giant papillary conjunctivitis induced by hard and soft contact lens wear: Quantitative histology. *Ophthalmology* 1979; 85:766.
5. Dvorak HF, Dvorak AM, Simpson BA, et al: Cutaneous basophil hypersensitivity. II. A light and electron microscopic description. *J Exp Med* 1970; 132:558.
6. Meiser DM, Krachmer JH, Goeker JA: An immunopathologic study of giant papillary conjunctivitis associated with ocular prostheses. *Am J Ophthalmol* 1981; 92:368.
7. Ponshik PC, Ballow M: Tear immunoglobulins in giant papillary conjunctivitis induced by contact lenses. *Am J Ophthalmol* 1983; 96:460.
8. Allansmith MR: Summary and conclusion, in Lass JH (ed): *The First Cromolyn Sodium in Ophthalmology.* Princeton, NJ, Excerta Medica, 1985, pp 34–35.
9. Korb DR, Greiner JV, Finnemore VM, et al: Treatment of contact lenses with papain. Increase in wearing time in keratoconus patients with papillary conjunctivitis. *Arch Ophthalmol* 1983; 101:48.

Cylinders and Bifocals—When to Put on an Addition?

APPROACH 1

Benjamin Milder, M.D.

APPROACH 2

David L. Guyton, M.D.

Case 21

Cylinders and Bifocals—When to Put on an Addition?

A 43-year-old bookkeeper presents because of difficulty reading through her glasses. Her present glasses are $-2.00 + 1.75 \times 90$ in each eye. Her new refraction is $-2.50 + 1.75 \times 105 = 20/15$ and $-2.50 + 1.75 \times 75 = 20/15$, requiring $+1.00$ D more to see 4-point print comfortably.

Should the cylinder axis be changed at this point, and what bifocal should be ordered?

Summary _____

Refraction and prescribing are central to general ophthalmology, and decision making is usually straightforward. However, there are some common situations in which the refractionist is often left wondering which course of action is best. That is the situation in the case of this 43-year-old woman with a changing cylinder and a new need for help at the near position.

After arguing in favor of prescribing the cylinder at the correct axis, Dr. Milder discusses which type of bifocal he would recommend for this patient. He concludes that she would be best served with progressive addition lenses.

In his discussion of the bifocal correction, Dr. Guyton advocates prescribing a $+1.25$ D add because he believes that patients adjust to their first pair of bifocals more rapidly if this amount is used than if a smaller correction is given.

Both of the discussants stress the importance of allowing the patient to "test-drive" the distance correction in the office by using a trial frame. While this will not always discover patients who absolutely cannot tolerate a change in cylinder power or axis, it should reduce the frequency with which prescriptions have to be changed 2 weeks after they are written.

Approach 1 ⎯⎯⎯⎯⎯⎯⎯⎯⎯⎯⎯⎯⎯⎯

Benjamin Milder, M.D.

Corrective lenses should always address the patient's chief complaint—in this case, difficulty in reading vision. The refractionist is confronted by two problems here: (1) the change in cylinder axis as compared with the old glasses and (2) the amount of add (or no add).

The Cylinder Axis

Generally, maximum visual acuity is achieved by prescribing the refractive findings, i.e., the cylinder axis found at the new refraction.

The visual acuity with the old glasses is not provided. However, with a cylinder power of 1.75 D, one can expect that the acuity is compromised when the axes are 15 degrees off from the actual refraction. An axis error of this amount with a 1.75 D cylinder power would generate a new cylinder of approximately 0.75 D with its axis 45 degrees away from the midpoint between the true cylinder and the cylinder error. Thus, if the cylinder axis is 75 degrees and the lens is placed at axis 90 degrees, a new cylinder at axis 37.5 degrees would reduce visual acuity by 1 to 2 lines on the Snellen chart.[1]

In this patient, since the cylinder power is the same for the two eyes, unchanged from the old glasses, and since the deflection of cylinder axis from axis 90 degrees is symmetrical for the two eyes (105 and 75 degrees, respectively), adaptation to this new prescription should be rapid and uneventful.

It is helpful to place the new refraction findings in a trial frame, have the patient read and move about, and listen (without prompting the patient) for any complaints. If none are volunteered, I would prescribe the cylinder axes as found in the refraction.

If the patient is unable to tolerate the new correction in a trial frame, the appropriate course of action would be to demonstrate the decrease in visual acuity when reverting to the old axis so that the patient will be aware of the compromise in vision. In my opinion, prescribing the old axes should be reserved for the patient who has clearly demonstrated an inability to adapt to the actual refractive correction.

It must be remembered that the clinician is treating a patient and not just a pair of eyes. Careful history taking, careful observation of the patient, and attention to the patient's responses during the refraction will provide clues to the occasional patient who may be intolerant of change. There is no logic in routinely and arbitrarily selecting a prescription other than that found at refraction unless the patient has a prior history of intolerance to change or demonstrates an inability to adapt to the new prescription within a reasonable period of time—10 to 15 days.

In order to reduce the adaptation time with the new glasses, it is important to maintain without change those lens design characteristics that could lead, unnecessarily, to image size changes. Base curves, center thicknesses, vertex distance, and frame size should match the old glasses as closely as possible.[2]

The Reading Add Power

The visual acuity with the old glasses is not given, but the patient had no complaint regarding distance vision, and therefore it can be assumed that, although the old glasses represent + 0.50 D overcorrection for distance, this is not a source of trouble. The old glasses provide the equivalent of a + 0.50 D add, but since the patient has problems reading with the old prescription, it is apparent that she does, in fact, require additional add power for comfortable near vision.

Let us analyze this recommendation. Since the near vision measurements with the old glasses are not supplied, we must make several reasonable assumptions.

Assumption 1

At the age of 43, the patient should have approximately 4 D of accommodative amplitude.

Assumption 2

The patient should be able to use one half of that amplitude with comfort (a precarious assumption, but let us use it for the moment). Therefore, since the old glasses were overcorrected by 0.50 D, the patient should have been able to read comfortably at 40 cm by using 2 D of her accommodation plus the 0.5 D overcorrection.

Since the patient is not comfortable with the old glasses, it must be concluded that (1) accommodation is subnormal; (2) she cannot sustain that level of accommodation, or (3) her working distance must be shorter than 40 cm. The actual difficulty may be any one or combination of these three.

Assumption 3

The lady is short (say, less than 5 feet, 2 inches tall), and therefore her comfortable reading distance is actually 33 to 35 cm (requiring 3 D of accommodation).

Dilemma

With the old glasses at a natural comfort distance of 33 cm, the patient would be stressing her accommodation. At 40 cm, she would be more comfortable but would lose magnification. Since she does, in fact, have a near-vision complaint, either or both of these problems must be present. To avoid losing magnification or overstressing her accommodation, she will need the + 1.00 D reading add.

What about simply removing the glasses for near vision? The new refraction yields a spherical equivalent of − 1.50 D so that omitting the glasses would provide the equivalent of a + 1.50 D add with a far point of 67 cm. Omitting the glasses would sacrifice some intermediate range acuity as well as usable distance vision.

Furthermore, the absent 1.75 D correction for astigmatism would mean loss of acuity, with vision being reduced to between 80% and 85% visual efficiency. This is an unnecessary loss of vision. If the eye attempts to improve its resolving power by accommodating so that one end of the conoid of Sturm falls on the retina, symptoms of low-grade accommodative spasm could be added to the reduced acuity. For both of these reasons and since the goal of the refractionist is to maximize vision and relieve symptoms, reading without glasses is not an acceptable alternative.

Recommendation

Prescribe the manifest findings; add +1.00 D.

Type of Multifocal

This prescription can be executed in a 28-mm flat-topped bifocal. Alternatively, since the patient must, in any case, adapt to a new spectacle-wearing experience, she would be a good candidate for progressive addition lenses. There are three good reasons for preferring progressives in this case:

1. Cosmesis should be considered.
2. With a minimal difference between the distance and near corrections in early presbyopia, there will be only minimal distortion in the lens periphery due to the inherent adventitious astigmatism encountered in these lenses. The patient will make a rapid adaptation in her working situation—as rapid as would be the case with flat-topped bifocals worn for the first time.
3. There will be no abrupt image jump as the direction of gaze passes down from the distance portion of the lens into the reading area.

In consideration of the fact that the patient is a member of the work force, presumably in contact with other workers and with the public, and in order to minimize the trauma of coming to grips with the stark reality of having reached the age of presbyopia, I would recommend the progressive addition lenses for this patient.

References

1. Guyton, DL: Prescribing cylinders: The problem of distortion. *Surv Ophthalmol* 1977; 22:177–188.
2. Milder B, Rubin MR: *The Fine Art of Prescribing Glasses Without Making a Spectacle of Yourself.* Gainesville, Fla, Triad, 1979, p 83.

Approach 2 ──────────────

David L. Guyton, M.D.

I generally prescribe the full cylinder at the correct axis unless there is evidence from a walking-around trial with trial frames or from an actual attempt at wearing glasses that the patient cannot tolerate the resulting binocular spatial distortion. Having the patient move about accentuates the awareness of any spatial distortion that is present. Also using full-aperture (38 mm) trial lenses rather than the more modern ones with smaller apertures allows a better test of the peripheral vision effects of the prospective glasses. Even so, walking-around trials are not always reliable!

In this case I would thus prescribe the actual refractive findings and assume that the patient passes a walking-around trial while being careful to warn her of the spatial distortion that she will experience before she adjusts to the glasses over a week or two. I would stress that she *will* adapt if she is patient enough and will see all the more clearly by doing so. Warning and encouragement are in order when prescribing *any* new pair of glasses, especially with a change in cylinder power or axis.

For academic purposes, one can also approach this case analytically. First, how much residual astigmatism will the patient be left with if the cylinders and axes of the old glasses are *not* changed to the new refraction? If the cylinder power (C) of a spectacle lens is correct but the axis is wrong by θ degrees, the residual astigmatism is equal to $2C \sin \theta$.[1, 2] In this case the patient will be left with $2(1.75) \sin 15$ degrees, or 0.91 D of residual astigmatism in each eye. This amount of residual astigmatism, almost 1 D, determines the amount of blur the patient will experience. Even if the cylinder power is reduced to the optimal value at the incorrect axes ($C \cos 2\theta = 1.52$ D), the residual astigmatism will still be C sin 2θ = 0.87 D,[1,2] enough to make a noticeable difference in visual acuity.

If the new refraction is prescribed for each eye, however, what problems is the patient likely to experience from binocular spatial distortion? Large cylinders with symmetrically disposed axes 15 degrees from the vertical are generally not tolerated if the patient has never worn astigmatic correction. Such is not the case with this patient, however, for the full-cylinder power is already in the glasses, albeit at the wrong axes. The patient has presumably fully adapted to the old glasses, so any change in binocular spatial perception will be due to the astigmatic difference between the new glasses and the old ones.[3] The astigmatic difference, including axis difference, will have to be calculated trigonometrically unless the axes have remained the same or unless overrefraction techniques were used to determine the new refraction. Trigonometric formulas for calculating the entire spherocylindrical difference between two refractions were first published by Naylor in 1968.[4] In the present case, such calculations reveal that changing the old glasses to the actual refractive findings will be equivalent to adding the following lenses to the old glasses:

$$RE = -0.95 + 0.91 \times 127.5$$
$$LE = -0.95 + 0.91 \times 52.5$$

These symmetrically oblique cylinders will cause definite spatial distortion if the patient's peripheral fusion is intact. (Distortion produced by cylinders is rarely if ever a problem in the absence of binocular vision, for it is the stereoscopic space sense under binocular conditions that greatly exaggerates the effects of small monocular image tilts or distortions caused by cylinders in spectacle lenses.[1] Isolated vertical lines may appear to tilt toward the patient. She may have the sensation of walking along the crest of a hill with the floor slanting away on both sides. Whether or not she will tolerate this spatial distortion is a matter of individual sensitivity to oblique aniseikonia, best judged empirically by a walking-around trial with the new correction in trial frames.

For reading, the patient will need bifocals or a separate pair of reading glasses. If a patient is already used to wearing glasses,

I recommend going to bifocals instead of switching between two pairs of glasses. It is possible that patient could read without her glasses, but unless she had discovered this herself and was comfortable doing so, I would not encourage it. The astigmatism is too great to permit clear vision if left uncorrected, and the switching back and forth between cylinder and no cylinder can cause prolonged difficulty in adapting to the new glasses. As for the amount of reading add to prescribe, I follow the teaching of not prescribing less than a +1.25 D add on the basis that this much difference between the top and bottom segments is necessary for the patient to distinguish between the focus provided by the two segments and allow rapid adjustment to using the bifocals for the first time.[5]

In summary, I would prescribe the full cylinder at the correct axis for the distance correction, that is, if the patient tolerates a walking-around trial, and provide warning and encouragement about distortion problems and adapting to them. I would also prescribe +1.25 D sphere reading adds.

References

1. Guyton DL: Prescribing cylinders: The problem of distortion. *Surv Ophthalmol* 1977; 22:177–188.
2. Del Priore LV, Guyton DL: The Jackson cross cylinder: A reappraisal. *Ophthalmology* 1986; 93:1461–1465.
3. Guyton DL: Prescribing cylinders postoperatively, in Ernest JT (ed): *The Year Book of Ophthalmology—1985.* Chicago, Year Book Medical Publishers, Inc, 1985, pp 63–66.
4. Naylor EJ: Astigmatic difference in refractive errors. *Br J Ophthalmol* 1968; 52:422–425.
5. Sloane AE, Garcia GE: *Manual of Refraction*, ed 3. Boston, Little, Brown & Co, Inc, 1979, p 135.

SECTION *VIII*

Extraocular and Periocular Surgery

Case 22

Secondary Exotropia— How Best to Correct?

APPROACH 1

Eugene R. Folk, M.D.

APPROACH 2

Ronald V. Keech, M.D.
William E. Scott, M.D.

Case 22 _____

Secondary Exotropia—How Best to Correct?

A 20-year-old woman presents with exotropia. She had had muscle surgery on each eye at the age of 3 for esotropia but for the past few years had noticed an increasing exodeviation.

The visual acuity is 20/40 in the right eye and 20/20 in the left without correction. A cycloplegic refraction achieves the same acuities with a moderate hyperopic correction. She has a 30 prism diopter constant exotropia at near and distance.

The patient would like to have an improved cosmetic appearance.

Summary

Most strabismus surgery for esotropia is done on children, and while short-term results are excellent when using a variety of approaches, the late development of secondary exotropia commonly occurs. This young lady has developed such a deviation that it is cosmetically unacceptable to her.

Dr. Folk emphasizes the importance of evaluating the action of the medial recti prior to deciding on the best surgical approach. If there is poor medial rectus function, the surgery is aimed at strengthening the medial rectus with a resection and advancement to the area of the original insertion.

A recess/resect operation is advocated by Drs. Keech and Scott. While the approach to the medial rectus is similar to that of Dr. Folk (a resection and/or advancement), the magnitude is smaller, and this allows a concomitant recession of the lateral rectus. The lateral is placed on an adjustable suture, and the patient is left slightly overcorrected.

This complication of childhood surgery is common and can occur decades after the original procedure. Both of these approaches can be expected to give excellent results when the correct procedure is selected for the patient's particular deviation pattern.

Approach 1 _____

Eugene R. Folk, M.D.

Secondary exotropia following surgery for a previously esotropic deviation is fairly common. As in the 20-year-old woman who presented in this case, the exotropia may not become manifested until many years after successful esotropia surgery.

There are a number of approaches to the problem of secondary exotropia. The patient should be reassured that this is a correctable condition. The patient is also concerned that the result of further surgery will not "hold" as occurred previously. It is important to reassure the patient that not only is the deviation correctable but that in all probability the deviation will not deteriorate.

For the most part, secondary exotropia is a surgical condition. These patients respond poorly to antisuppression training and diplopia awareness training. They generally have a fairly significant scotoma both on the esotropic and exotropic side of their deviations. This is fortunate for the ophthalmologist because postoperative diplopia is a relatively rare complication. In the early stages, overcorrecting myopic lenses can temporarily be helpful. However, the adult patient can rarely tolerate significant overcorrection. Nor are such corrections as effective as they would be in the immediately overcorrected child.

I like to break down the patients with secondary exotropia into two major categories: those with good medial rectus function and those with poor medial rectus function. In general, the Urist-version light reflex test helps to differentiate the two groups of patients. Those patients who have 24 degrees or less of medial rotation are considered to have poor medial rectus function, and those who have better than 24 degrees of medial rotation are considered to have good medial rectus function.

304

Good Medial Rectus Function

Those patients who have good medial rectus function and have had surgery on one eye generally will benefit from surgery on the unoperated eye. Surgery is much more predictable when it is performed on eyes that have not had previous surgery. If the initial procedure is a large lateral rectus recession or recess-resect on the right eye, I would think that the procedure of choice would be a surgical procedure on the left eye. With the amount of deviation indicated here, I would be inclined to do an 8-mm recession of the left lateral rectus and an 8-mm resection of the left medial rectus. I would put the lateral rectus on an adjustable suture.

If the previous surgery had been a bilateral medial rectus recession, the procedure of choice in my hands would be a bilateral lateral rectus recession of 8-mm. Again, I would prefer operating on muscles that have not had previous surgery. In a 20-year-old patient, I would routinely place one of the laterals on an adjustable suture. If one does a unilateral lateral rectus recession in a patient who has had bilateral medial rectus recessions, the cosmetic effect is most unpleasant. There is a definite asymmetry of the palpebral fissures, with the eye having a recession of both recti having the wider palpebral fissure with some mild proptosis. This is caused by the releasing action of a recessed medial and lateral rectus.

If the patient had previous surgery on the horizontal muscles of both eyes, the corrective surgery would probably best be done on the deviating eye. If there was no clear-cut deviating eye, I would repeat the surgery on the eye that showed the least side effects from the previous operations. In other words, if there was a great deal of granulation or scar tissue over one muscle in one eye, I would be inclined to do any further surgery on the other eye, perhaps excising the scar tissue from the affected eye at the same time. Here, again, the procedure of choice is to do a total of 8 mm of surgery on the medial rectus muscle. In other words, if the muscle is found to have previous 5-mm recession, I would advance the medial 5 mm and resect 3 mm. If previous surgery consisted of a 4-mm recession, I would advance the medial 4 mm and resect 4 mm. I would recess the conjunctiva over the medial rectus at this time to minimize the scar tissue. At the same time I would recess the lateral in the affected eye a total of 8 mm and put that muscle on an adjustable suture. As part of my adjustable-suture technique, I would recess the conjunctiva. Thus, the conjunctiva over both the medial and lateral recti in the operated eye would be recessed. This is an important feature because reoperations do produce more scar tissue and the patients are aware of this once they have overcome the initial pleasure of having straight eyes. Thus, we can see that in the patient who has a secondary exotropia with good medial rectus function three options are available for the correction of the deviation.

Poor Medial Rectus Function

In the patient who has poor medial rectus function, the surgical procedure of choice is a large resection and advancement of the affected medial rectus muscle. Until that underacting muscle is corrected, the patient will always show a significant deviation in the field of action of that medial rectus muscle. This can only be corrected with surgery on the muscle itself. We have found that the resection and advancement operation on an underacting medial rectus muscle is a very powerful operation, can easily correct the amount of deviation the patient demonstrates, and in many cases will correct 30 to 40 prism diopters of secondary exotropia. A limbal approach is made and the muscle picked up on a muscle hook. Careful dissection of the surrounding check ligaments and intermuscular membranes has to be done so that the medial rectus is cleaned as far back as possible. One should attempt to do at least an 8-mm resection as well as an advancement to a position about 5 mm from the limbus. Usually a fair amount of scar tissue is encountered, and this scar tissue should be excised once the muscle has been reattached to its new insertion. Failure to excise this scar tissue results in probably the worst-looking scar of any type of motility surgery. It is wise to excise some of the thick capsule that is usually present as well. The conjunctiva is then recessed to the new medial rectus insertion. This will allow 5 mm of bare sclera between the new insertion and the limbus.

In this manner a scar forms that is quite satisfactory. A recession of the lateral rectus opposite the large resection and advancement is usually not warranted and can frequently lead to overcorrections. With the large resection and advancement, the lateral rectus cannot be put on an adjustable suture. The medial rectus is so tight the first couple of days that it is impossible to pull up the lateral to compensate for an overcorrection. As a result, when we find a patient who has an underacting medial rectus with a secondary exotropia, surgery is limited to that resection and advancement of that medial rectus muscle. If the deviation is over 40 prism diopters, both medials have had surgery, and both medials are underacting, this procedure can be performed on both medial rectus muscles. However, you should have over 40 prism diopters of deviation because it is easy to overcorrect with this very powerful operation.

In summary, therefore, secondary exotropia is correctable. It is common. It can occur many years after the original esotropia surgery. Criteria to be watched for are underaction of the medial rectus muscle and abnormalities of the palpebral fissure.

Approach 2 _____

Ronald V. Keech, M.D.
William E. Scott, M.D.

The case presented is a 20-year-old woman who underwent esotropia surgery as a child and sometime later developed a 30 prism
diopter exotropia. Exodeviations following surgery for esotropia
have been reported in the literature to occur between 4.6% and
20% of the time. The frequency varies with the selection criteria.
Studies with higher rates generally cite all overcorrections following esotropia surgery. Others consider only exodeviations greater
than 10 prism diopters and report a correspondingly lower overcorrection rate. Another factor is the length of follow-up. Most
experts agree that the longer the follow-up period, the greater the
number of overcorrections.

The cause of overcorrections from esotropia surgery is not well
understood. Some authors attribute the problem to an inadequate
evaluation or to excessive surgery. Others point to the presence
of A or V patterns, vertical deviation, and amblyopia as important
contributing factors. Still other experts attribute the cause to an
indirect effect upon the convergence center and the natural decrease in accommodative convergence with age.

Evaluation

In this case, as with any reoperation, the strabismus surgeon
must carefully look for any factors that may affect the success of
an additional procedure. A good history of the previous esotropia
would be useful. While not essential, this information might distinguish between an infantile esotropia with poor fusional poten-

tial and an acquired, partially accommodative esotropia with a better prognosis for fusion.

As much data as possible should be attained about the previous procedure. It is likely that this patient had bilateral medial rectus recessions, but perhaps three or four muscles were operated on. The surgery record may detail any anomalous muscle insertions, unusual difficulties, or unexpected procedures such as a muscle transposition. This information will help in estimating the amount of time and difficulty required for the reoperation.

The examination provides the most valuable information for planning treatment. A careful evaluation of the ocular deviation in the cardinal positions of gaze is indicated in all surgical candidates but is especially important with reoperations. Excessive muscle surgery may create restrictions or weakness. This can be demonstrated by the presence of an incomitant deviation, abnormal versions, or positive forced ductions. A marked lateral gaze incomitance may also occur without obvious muscle restriction or weakness. A significant incomitancy should be corrected at the time of surgery to reduce the risk of increased postoperative instability.

The sensory status is less important than motor alignment but can provide useful information. A good fusional response may suggest a more stable postoperative alignment. Location of suppression scotomas should also be documented. This can help in advising the patient about postoperative diplopia.

The refractive error is another important factor that must be considered in the treatment of strabismus. The effect of accommodation on a deviation can be significant. The exodeviation in the case under consideration could increase with correction of the "moderate hyperopia." With normal uncorrected vision in her left eye, however, it is unlikely that this patient would wear glasses. Therefore, we would prefer to operate for the deviation measured without correction of the refractive error.

Treatment

A moderate or large exodeviation is best treated with surgery.

If further evaluation of this case indicates a basic exodeviation with no other variables, we would perform a recession-resection procedure on the amblyopic right eye. The medical rectus muscle would be explored and advanced or resected approximately 6 mm. The lateral rectus would be recessed 8 mm on an adjustable suture with a plan to advance the muscle postoperatively if necessary. The adjustable suture provides a method to refine the initial postoperative alignment and to avoid gross overcorrections or undercorrections.

We would prefer to overcorrect this patient 4 to 14 prism diopters at the time of adjustment with perhaps a very mild restriction to abduction initially. In our experience, the likelihood of a permanent overcorrection is low. In our last 23 cases of secondary exotropia following esotropia surgery, 15 of the patients had an exodrift postoperatively, 4 had an esodrift, and 4 remain unchanged from their postadjustment alignment.

The surgical plan would be modified according to any additional findings found on the examination. For example, if the patient had moderate to marked limitation to adduction of the left eye due to decreased medial rectus function or a tight lateral rectus, we would operate on that eye. If the sensory evaluation revealed both nasal and temporal suppression, we would prefer to overcorrect less in order to avoid a recurrence of the esotropia.

Under selected conditions, we would consider an Oculinum injection as an alternate treatment for this type of deviation. Oculinum or botulinum toxin has been used for a number of years under a Food and Drug Administration (FDA) approved investigation protocol for the treatment of strabismus. It functions by paralyzing the treated muscle for a few weeks to months, thus allowing contraction of the antagonist muscle. The ability of botulinum to change the ocular alignment is well documented. Less certain is the predictability and permanence of the effect and the unintentional involvement of other ocular muscles such as the levator. Repeated injections also are often necessary for moderate or large deviations.

In summary, we would perform a recession and resection procedure on the amblyopic right eye of this patient by using an adjustable suture technique. The patient would be left slightly esotropic following the adjustment. If she were reluctant to undergo surgery or had contraindications to anesthesia, we would recommend treatment with botulinum.

Bibliography

1. Cooper ED: The surgical management of secondary exotropia. *Trans Am Acad Ophthalmol Otolaryngol* 1961; 65:595–601.
2. Yazawa K: Postoperative exotropia. *J Pediatr Ophthalmol* 1981; 18:58–64.
3. Keech RV, Scott WE, Christensen LE: Adjustable suture strabismus surgery. *J Pediatr Ophthalmol Strabismus* 1987; 24:97–102.
4. Scott AB: Botulinum toxin injection of eye muscles to correct strabismus. *Trans Am Ophthalmol Soc* 1981; 79:734–770.

Case 23 —————————————

Chalazia—Soak, Poke, or Cut?

APPROACH 1

Frederick A. Jakobiec, M.D.
I. Rand Rodgers, M.D.

APPROACH 2

Jeffery B. Robin, M.D.

Case 23

Chalazia—Soak, Poke, or Cut?

A 59-year-old man has had four chalazia excised from his eyelids over the past 6 years. He now presents with a chalazion in his left lower lid. He wishes to be rid of the lesion, but asks if there are any modalities available aside from surgical excision.

What alternatives are possible?

Summary _____

Chalazia are an extremely common clinical problem in general ophthalmology, and both patients and physicians are interested in nonsurgical alternatives. This patient has had several chalazia excised in the past few years and is anxious to find a choice other than the pain and inconvenience of excision.

Intralesion steroid injection, a technique pioneered in their practice, is advocated by Drs. Jakobiec and Rodgers. This approach would seem to satisfy the patient's desire to avoid "surgery," while presenting an alternative with a reported success rate of over 70%. The authors stress the side effects of this treatment, particularly the development of hypopigmented spots over the site of injection.

Dr. Robin, after reviewing the clinical and pathogenetic characteristics of chalazia, advocates surgical excision. He points out that, despite the patient's wishes to the contrary, there is a risk that the lesion represents a recurrence of an old "chalazion." Such a lesion should be assumed to be malignant until biopsy proves it otherwise. A careful explanation of this problem is likely to convince the patient that excisional biopsy is in his best interest.

Both discussions stress that conservative management with hot compresses is likely to result in resolution of early chalazia. They both also stress that a recurrent chalazion should arouse suspicion of a malignancy and that that suspicion should trigger a decision to perform a biopsy of the lesion.

Approach 1 _____

Frederick A. Jakobiec, M.D.
I. Rand Rodgers, M.D.

Occlusion of a sebaceous gland duct within either the upper or lower eyelid commences the pathophysiological process whereby acute and chronic inflammatory eyelid lesions develop. An internal hordeolum or chalazion is characterized by acute erythema and tenderness over an obstructed meibomian or Zeis gland; the contents of the chalazion are generally devoid of an infectious agent. If untreated or if recalcitrant to treatment, a firm, minimally tender mass will develop. Such a mass may perforate the tarsus to envelope anterior lamellar structures or rupture through the conjunctiva to form a polypoid mass, sometimes associated with an overlying pyogenic granuloma. When excised and examined under the light microscope, confluent series of focal granulomas, multinucleated giant cells, neutrophils, lymphocytes, and plasma cells are observed to be dispersed amid lipid globules. Asteroid and Schaumann bodies are occasionally present.[1] Treatments besides surgical excision include warm compresses, antibiotics, and intralesional steroid injections. Antibiotics are employed in case a low-grade conjunctivitis has contributed to the blockage of the ostia of the meibomian gland ducts. The choice of treatment modality is influenced by the patient's desire, age, and findings suspicious for a masquerade syndrome, which is usually a sebaceous carcinoma.

The external hordeolum, or stye, results from a purulent inflammation of the follicle of a cilium and the glands of Zeis. Warm compresses are the recommended treatment. Applied 4 to 5 times per day for 5 to 10 minutes each, warm compresses promote blood supply to the affected gland and dilation of its obstructed orifice.

Antibiotic ointment applied to the skin or topical drops may supplement the aforementioned regimen. For those patients with severe inflammation or discomfort or those concerned by their cosmesis, incision and drainage of such lesions is reasonable. Local anesthesia is attained and an incision made over the fluctuant region. Postdrainage warm compresses should be continued.

Chalazia tend to be chronic inflammatory lesions that may persist for months or resolve spontaneously with or without recurrence. Warm compresses applied 4 to 5 times a day for 5 to 10 minutes each is the accepted initial treatment for patients of all age groups. Again, if the patient finds the lesion cosmetically disfiguring and desires surgery, it should be done.

Intralesional steroid injection or surgery is generally reserved for those chalazia that do not regress with warm compresses. Steroids suppress the inflammatory cell response and impede chronic fibrosis and scar formation. Leinfelder[2] was the first to successfully treat chalazia with steroids. He injected 0.25 mL of methylprednisolone acetate subconjunctivally in the quadrant containing the chalazia to convert acute and chronic chalazia into more compact lesions. Pizzarello et al.[3] directly injected chalazia with a long-acting steroid. Of 17 chalazia injected, 13 displayed prompt and lasting resolution within 1 to 2 weeks after one or two injections. Two lesions did not subside at all, while 2 others recurred. Mohan et al.[4] found the response to intralesional steroids to be unrelated to the duration of symptoms. Two thirds of the rock-hard chalazia in their study resolved completely after steroid injection, thus lending speculation that the firm consistency is not necessarily due to fibrosis but rather to tense swelling of the capsule.

The advantages of intralesional injection of steroids are myriad. Technically a simple procedure, it subjects the patients to a minimum of pain or discomfort. The risk of damage to the canaliculi and eyelid margin by surgery is eliminated, and rarely is there any blood loss. It furthermore spares young children the need for and risk of a general anesthetic. Complications are rare. Cutaneous atrophy and depigmentation in blacks and darkly pigmented individuals have been reported, but if the lesion is injected from the conjunctival side, these complications are less likely to occur. Recently, a retinal and choroidal vascular occlusion following intralesional steroid injection was reported,[5] but this is exceedingly uncommon. Injection of the steroid material into an artery with retrograde flow toward the eyeball under pressure may account for this complication; lesions of the eyelid margin or supratarsal regions next to the vascular arcades of the eyelids (terminal branches of the ophthalmic artery) probably should not be treated by injection.

We recommend intralesional injection of 0.05 to 0.3 mL of triamcinolone acetate, 5 mg/mL suspension, for chalazia unresponsive to warm compresses. Direct injection into the chalazion may be difficult because of the unyielding framework of the tarsus. Therefore, injection in a pretarsal plane beneath the orbicularis muscle may be necessary and is efficacious since the steroidal material can diffuse. For large chalazia repeat injections may be required. If after multiple injections the chalazion does not resolve, excisional biopsy and histopathologic studies are performed to rule out a masquerade lesion. Intralesional steroids will not result in a dramatic short-term response if a meibomian gland neoplasm is present. For older patients with a history of chronic conjunctivitis, blepharitis, and "chalazia," a full-thickness eyelid biopsy is performed to rule out a sebaceous gland carcinoma.

For this 59-year-old gentleman who presents with a left lower-lid mass we recommend a trial of warm compresses. If the mass does not subsequently resolve, an intralesional triamcinolone acetate injection would be our preferred treatment. If after multiple injections the mass does not regress, it should be excised and submitted for pathological examination.

References

1. Font RL: Eyelids and lacrimal drainage system, in Spencer WH (ed): *Ophthalmic Pathology: An Atlas and Textbook*, vol 3, ed 3. Philadelphia, WB Saunders Co, 1986, pp 2266–2268.
2. Leinfelder PJ: Depo-Medrol in treatment of acute chalazion. *Am J Ophthalmol* 1964; 58:1078–1081.
3. Pizzarello LD, Jakobiec FA, Hofeldt AJ, et al: Intralesional corticosteroid therapy of chalazia. *Am J Ophthalmol* 1978; 85:818–821.

4. Mohan K, Dhir SP, Munjal VP, et al: The use of intralesional steroids in the treatment of chalazion. *Ann Ophthalmol* 1986; 18:158–160.

5. Thomas EL, Laborde RP: Retinal and choroidal vascular occlusion following intralesional corticosteroid injection of a chalazion. *Ophthalmology* 1986; 93:405–407.

Approach 2 ─────────────────────────

Jeffrey B. Robin, M.D.

This case is that of a 59-year-old man with a history of recurrent chalazia that have been treated with surgical excision. It is not specified whether or not the lesions have been unilateral or bilateral. Additionally, the race of the patient is not specified. The patient presents with a new chalazion involving the left lower lid. This discussion will be aimed at providing an overview of treatment options available in this condition. A thorough review of treatment options for chalazia should, however, be prefaced by a brief discussion of their clinical characteristics, pathogenesis, and differential diagnosis.

Clinical Characteristics and Demographics

Chalazia are probably the most commonly occurring lesions that involve the eyelids. They are chronic granulomatous inflammations originating in the meibomian glands and involving the surrounding eyelid tissues. Clinically, chalazia are characterized by the presence of a slowly progressive, discrete, firm, nontender mass. Their presence may follow acute inflammatory episodes of the meibomian glands.

Chalazia may occur in all age groups, from young children to the elderly. There is no known sex predilection for these lesions, nor is there a predilection for lesion location (left or right eye, upper or lower eyelid). It is not uncommon for patients with chalazia to also have a history of anterior blepharitis, meibomian gland dysfunction (MGD), and/or acne rosacea. Patients with small chalazia are generally asymptomatic; as the lesions grow in size, patients generally will complain of the cosmetic disfigurement. Uncommonly, large chalazia may compress the peripheral cornea and result in the induction of irregular astigmatism with perceptible visual distortion.

According to Duke-Elder, chalazia may be clinically classified by their location within the eyelid. Chalazion internum, or a deep chalazion, occurs adjacent to the conjunctival surface. Chalazion externum, or a superficial chalazion, occurs in the anterior portions of the eyelid closer to the skin surface. A marginal chalazion primarily involves the eyelid margin.

Pathogenesis

Chalazia are chronic granulomatous inflammatory reactions occurring in the vicinity of the meibomian glands of the eyelids. Histopathologically, they are characterized by zonal granulomatous inflammation centered around the lipid deposits that have extruded from the glands into the surrounding eyelid tissue. The affected tissue contains a multitude of foreign-body (Langhans') giant cells plus chronic inflammatory cells that form a typical granuloma pattern. Occasionally, bacteria may be found within the area of the granulomatous reaction.

The meibomian glands produce the lipid layer of the tear film. They are holocrine glands, having secretions that are composed in part of desquamated epithelial cells from the ductal linings plus released cytoplasmic contents rich in lipids. Dysfunction of the meibomian glands is a relatively common clinical syndrome that can lead to rapid breakup of the tear film and subsequent "dry-eye" symptoms. MGD is almost invariably noted in patients who have acne rosacea, a chronic dysfunction of the lipid-producing sebaceous glands.

Because of the embryological similarity between the sebaceous and meibomian glands, investigators have used the known cause of sebaceous gland dysfunction (hyperkeratinization of the ductal epithelium that produces chronic obstruction) to examine the pathogenesis of MGD. Creating an experimental model of MGD, Jester and associates observed that hyperkeratinization of the ductal epithelium of the gland orifices did indeed occur and appeared to be the initiating event. Histopathological specimens from clinical cases of MGD have confirmed that hyperkeratinization of the ductal epithelium, primarily at the orifices, is a consistent feature and not uncommonly results in orifice obstruction. Additionally, in both the experimental model and clinical cases, dilation of the distal portions of the ducts of affected meibomian glands was commonly noted. Using transillumination and infrared photography, detailed in vivo examinations of meibomian gland morphology can be performed. Using this technique in experimental and clinical MGD confirmed that dilation of the distal ducts (particularly in those glands that were noted to have inspissated material in their orifices) was an important feature. In clinical cases of severe MGD, some of the glands were noted to have areas that had become completely sequestered; these areas corresponded clinically to yellowish deposits visible beneath the tarsal conjunctiva (sometimes referred to as "microchalazia").

Using the data and observations from experimental models of MGD as well as clinical cases of MGD, it appears that chalazia may represent the severe end of the MGD spectrum. The pathogenesis of chalazia, therefore, is most likely related to chronic obstruction of the meibomian gland orifices (from hyperkeratinization of the ductal epithelium) that produces dilation and eventual sequestration of distal portions of the ducts. The lipid from these sequestered portions eventually extrudes into surrounding eyelid tissue, which incites a foreign body type of granulomatous inflammatory response. A similar histopathologic response can be produced experimentally by injecting sterile mutton fat or yellow wax into eyelid tissues. No evidence to date has been produced that confirms any role for infection in the pathogenesis of chalazia.

Treatment

Small, cosmetically acceptable chalazia generally require no treatment. If there is a component of active eyelid inflammation, warm compresses and antibiotic ointments are indicated. Larger, more cosmetically objectionable chalazia can be treated with either incision and curettage or injection of corticosteroids.

Incision and Curettage

Surgical incision with curettage has been the mainstay of chalazion therapy. Local infiltration anesthesia, usually with a short-acting agent such as 1% xylocaine, is administered around the chalazion. Generally, epinephrine (1:100,000) is included in the anesthetic mixture to minimize bleeding. Any of a variety of chalazion clamps are then used to isolate the lesion and provide hemostasis. Depending upon whether the chalazion is deep or superficial, the lesion is approached from either the conjunctival or skin surfaces. A scalpel is then used to incise down to the capsule of the lesion. It is recommended to make conjunctival incisions vertically so that other meibomian glands will not be damaged. For incisions on the skin surface, a scleral shell should be used to protect the underlying globe. Once the capsule is identified, it is incised, and a curette is used to remove the contents of the lesion. Generally, healing can occur via secondary intention. Postoperatively, antibiotic ointment is applied and the eye is patched tightly for approximately 6 to 12 hours in order to ensure comfort and provide pressure for hemostasis.

The results of surgical therapy for chalazia are considered to be excellent. Complications, although rare, can occur; these include full-thickness penetration through the eyelid, injury to the underlying globe, infection, extensive hemorrhage into the eyelid, and even retrobulbar hemorrhage. Additionally, although the procedure is quite minor, for some patients (because of their age or level of apprehension) nonsurgical therapy may be preferable.

Corticosteroid Injection

The first report of corticosteroid injections for the treatment of chalazia was from Leinfelder in 1964. A suspension of methylprednisolone acetate (Depo-Medrol) was placed subconjunctivally adjacent to the lesion in order to decrease the inflammatory reaction. In some of the cases, this was followed by incision and curettage. In 1978, Pizzarello and associates reported the use of triamcinolone acetonide for chalazia. They injected a 5-mg/mL suspension of this agent directly into the lesion in 17 patients.

Complete resolution was noted in 13 (76%). Because this study was uncontrolled, a question emerged as to whether the clinical effect was indeed from the steroid or merely from the needle incision of the capsule and the subsequent injection-induced extrusion of the contents of the chalazion. In a randomly assigned group of patients, Sloas and colleagues treated chalazia with intralesional injections of either normal saline or triamcinolone acetonide (10 mg/mL). They found that, while 66% of the steroid-treated lesions resolved, none of the saline-injected lesions improved. Of the latter group, eight were eventually cured with subsequent triamcinolone injections.

It is apparent from the aforementioned studies that intralesional triamcinolone therapy is a viable alternative for those patients who do not respond to conservative therapy (warm compresses and antibiotics) and who do not wish to undergo incision and curettage. There are potential problems associated with steroid injection therapy. Patients may note significant pain upon injection. Postinjection, adverse effects upon the eyelids have been noted; these include hyperpigmentation, subcutaneous fat atrophy; and particularly in darker pigmented individuals, hypopigmentation. Additionally, periocular steroids have been associated with intraocular pressure elevations.

Recommendation

I approach the treatment of chalazia in the following manner. First-time chalazia in lightly pigmented patients are treated with intralesional triamcinolone (10 mg/mL). Because of the potential for hypopigmentation of the eyelid skin, darker-pigmented patients are treated with incision and curettage. Additionally, I look carefully for any signs of associated MGD and rosacea; affected patients are placed on regimens of oral tetracycline. I generally treat recurrent chalazia and those that have failed intralesional steroid therapy with incision and curettage. It is appropriate, at this point in the discussion, to strongly emphasize that recurrent or nonresponsive chalazia may not, in fact, be chalazia.

The major differential diagnostic consideration for a presumed chalazion is that of sebaceous gland carcinoma. The classic presentation of these potentially fatal lesions is that of a "recurring chalazion." These malignant tumors comprise 0.2% to 1.3% of all lid tumors but are the most malignant, with a mortality rate of 6% to 30%. They generally occur in older individuals, with an average age at diagnosis of 58 years; they have, however, been reported to occur as early as the age of 3 years. Sebaceous gland carcinomas more frequently affect females and, additionally, have a predilection for the upper eyelid. The fact that these carcinomas frequently resemble chalazia and other less aggressive lesions all too often results in delayed diagnosis. Clinical suspicion is probably the most important factor in reducing mortality rates. Therefore, recurrent or nonresponsive chalazia should have incision and curettage, with the removed material submitted for histopathologic evaluation.

In conclusion, the present case is that of a recurrent chalazion in the left lower eyelid of a 59-year-old male who desires an alternative to surgical intervention. In spite of the patient's concerns, I would recommend surgical incision with curettage and submission of material for histopathologic evaluation. Even though sebaceous gland carcinomas more commonly occur in females and more commonly involve the upper eyelid, the risk that this potentially fatal lesion poses far outweighs the convenience of alternative therapies. I have found that, if appropriately explained, most patients in this situation will readily accept the surgical option. The onus, in these cases, is certainly upon the ophthalmologist to maintain a sufficient level of clinical suspicion.

Bibliography

1. Cohen BZ, Tripathi RC: Eyelid depigmentation after intralesional injection of a fluorinated corticosteroid for chalazion. *Am J Ophthalmol* 1979; 88:269.
2. Duke Elder S (ed): *System of Ophthalmology*, vol 13. St Louis, CV Mosby Co, 1974.
3. Harvey JT, Anderson RL: The management of meibomian gland carcinoma. *Ophthalmic Surg* 1982; 13:56.
4. Jester JV, Nicolaides N, Smith RE: Meibomian gland studies: Histo-

logic and ultrastructural investigations. *Invest Ophthalmol Vis Sci* 1981; 20:537.

5. Jester JV, Rife L, Nii D, et al: In vivo biomicroscopy and photography of meibomian glands in a rabbit model of meibomian gland dysfunction. *Invest Ophthalmol Vis Sci* 1982: 22:660.

6. Leinfelder PJ: Depo-Medrol in treatment of acute chalazion. *Am J Ophthalmol* 1964; 58:1078.

7. Pizarello LD, Jakobiec FA, Hofeldt AJ, et al: Intralesional corticosteroid therapy of chalazia. *Am J Ophthalmol* 1978; 85:818.

8. Robin JB, Nobe J, Jester JV, et al: In vivo biomicroscopy of meibomian gland dysfunction: A clinical study. *Ophthalmology* 1985: 92:1423.

9. Sloas HA, Starling J, Galentin PG, et al: Treatment of chalazia with injectable triamcinolone. *Ann Ophthalmol* 1983; 15:78.

10. Wagoner MD, Beyer CK, Gonder JR, et al: Common presentations of sebaceous gland carcinoma of the eyelid. *Ann Ophthalmol* 1982; 14:159.

Acute Dacryocystitis— When Best to Operate?

APPROACH 1

Bartley R. Frueh, M.D.

APPROACH 2

John B. Holds, M.D.
Richard L. Anderson, M.D.

Case 24 _____

Acute Dacryocystitis—When Best to Operate?

A 58-year-old woman presents with acute dacry-ocystitis. She has had tearing for several years that has been managed with occasional irrigation, per-formed in the physician's office.

How should this attack be managed?

Summary _____

Patients of all ages develop nasolacrimal duct obstructions that can progress to acute dacryocystitis. The proper management of these cases, especially the timing of surgery, is the subject addressed in this case.

Dr. Frueh discusses techniques aimed at emptying the lacrimal sac. If the infection is not pointing to the skin, a Bowman probe can be placed into the sac, and pressure on the sac may allow it to empty. Percutaneous aspiration is also possible.

Drs. Holds and Anderson comment on the previous treatment that the patient received. Repeated irrigation only results in temporary relief and places the patient at risk for canalicular scarring that could jeopardize the success of a dacryocystorhinostomy (DCR) in the future.

Both authors counsel against DCR in the face of acute infection and inflammation. They both stress, however, that the patient should be encouraged to undergo DCR after 2 to 4 weeks because of the inevitability of future infections if surgery is withheld.

Approach 1 —————————————————

Bartley R. Frueh, M.D.

The history is that of an adult who has had tearing for several years and who has now developed acute dacryocystitis. I will assume that her tearing was only on one side, the same side that now has acute dacryocystitis. Since she is reported to have been managed in the past with occasional irrigations, performed in the physician's office, I will assume that, on those instances, irrigation fluid did pass into the nose and that she did experience relief of tearing, albeit temporary, following the irrigation. I will divide the discussion into the pathogenesis of her problem, management of the acute attack, and long-term management.

Pathogenesis

Since she initially had a functional obstruction that was temporarily relieved by irrigation, one of two things was occurring. She could have been developing a plug in her nasolacrimal duct that was forced out with the pressure of irrigation. We don't understand why these occur. It is supposed that they may be mucus plugs since in that case it would not be identified after it is out. Some people have firm casts form in their nasolacrimal duct that most commonly in my experience pass spontaneously, with pain during the moments they are passed, and there is recovery of the cast. I am not sure whether these casts represent inspissated mucus, in which case they would be a late form of a mucus cast, or other collected debris. More commonly, the patient would have formed a dacryolith, an accumulation of debris that in some but

330

not all cases is fungal in origin. I believe the pressure of irrigation dilates the sac around the dacryolith and permits fluid to go around it and into the nasolacrimal duct. I also suspect that the force of the irrigating fluid may change the position of the dacryolith sufficiently that fluid will go around it and give relief of tearing until it either becomes larger or shifts back to its previous position to reobstruct outflow.

To get acute dacryocystitis, one must have blockage of outflow and then have the tear sac contents become infected, with swelling blocking off backflow through the internal common punctum. With loss of egress of the infected contents, an abscess is formed that infects the surrounding tissue.

Management of Acute Dacryocystitis

Patients with acute dacryocystitis may be divided into two groups: those in which the tear sac abscess is pointing and those in which it is not. Both will have a tender, erythematous swelling over the area near the lacrimal crest, with cellulitis being evident. For the abscess to be pointing, it means the tissue between the tear sac and the skin has become very thin and may even open spontaneously and drain. It will usually be lighter in color in that area because the color of the pale pus is seen through the skin. Gentle palpation will reveal that the area is softer: being thinner, it is less indurated.

When the abscess is pointing, it should be incised, drained, and cultured just as one would treat any other pointing abscess. I prefer to incise with a pointed blade, such as a no. 11 Bard-Parker. This does not require local anesthesia: the tissue is too thin to infiltrate and is so tense that the patient will have little discomfort at the moment of incision and immense relief when the pressure of the abscess decreases with drainage. I prefer to express as much of the contents as possible and place a wick inside the sac through the incision. This keeps the wound open, allows further drainage, and prevents recurrence of the abscess.

When the abscess is not pointing, the pressure inside the sac should be relieved for the patient's comfort, to promote resolution of the infection, and to be able to culture the abscess. This can sometimes be accomplished by placing a small Bowman probe through the lower canaliculus and internal common punctum into the tear sac (about 14 mm). The probe is then pushed inferiorly, opening up the internal common punctum, while a little more pressure is placed on the sac. If this does not allow the sac to empty, the sac contents may be aspirated percutaneously. I find it best to use an 18-guage needle because the pus may be quite thick and thus not aspirate well with a smaller needle. A 5-cc syringe is usually adequate.

Patients with acute dacryocystitis should be treated with an appropriate systemic antibiotic after their sac is emptied and the contents Gram stained and cultured. This may often be done successfully as an outpatient, but hospital admission may be required if the infection is particularly virulent or the patient is immunocompromised so that intravenous antibiotics may be administered. I can think of no circumstance in which DCR should be performed during the acute infection.

Long-Term Management

Re-establishing tear drainage is necessary to eliminate the possibility of recurrence of infection. Definitive surgical therapy should be delayed until the cellulitis has cleared. I usually plan for DCR 3 to 4 weeks after the acute infection is treated. Because these acute infections are extremely painful, it is usually relatively easy to convince the patient that surgery should be performed to prevent a recurrence. While performing a DCR on this patient, it will be particularly important to inspect the sac for a dacryolith and remove any material that is found.

Approach 2 _____

John B. Holds, M.D.
Richard L Anderson, M.D.

Dacryocystitis arises as a result of a partial or complete blockage at the level of the nasolacrimal duct and permits tear stagnation, accumulation of cellular debris, and overgrowth of microorganisms within the lacrimal sac. The evaluation of the tearing patient is well outlined in numerous reference texts.[1-3] In acute dacryocystitis there is a complete blockage at the level of the nasolacrimal duct, and further functional testing is neither productive nor warranted. Nasolacrimal duct obstruction may be a result of congenital occlusion, trauma, tumors, dacryoliths, or nasal and sinus disease, but is most commonly idiopathic. Idiopathic nasolacrimal obstruction most frequently presents in midlife to latelife with a female-to-male preponderance variously reported from 4:1 to 9:1.[1, 4]

In adults, the most commonly reported organisms in acute dacryocystitis are *Staphylococcus aureus* or *Staphylococcus epidermidis*. *Streptococcus pneumoniae* is the next most common organism followed by *Hemophilus influenzae*.[5] Less common organisms include diphtheroids, *Klebsiella pneumoniae*, *Pseudomonas aeruginosa*, and rarely *Arachnia propionicum*, *Mycobacterium tuberculosis*, *Candida parapsilosis*, *Aspergillus niger*, and others.

The choice of initial antibiotic therapy in an adult with an otherwise unremarkable acute dacryocystitis is empirical. Cephalexin (Keflex), 500 mg orally four times daily, is effective against the most likely organisms listed earlier. Dicloxacillin (Dynapen), 500 mg orally four times daily, shows good activity against grampositive species including penicillinase-producing staphylococci.

A secondary agent is ampicillin, 500 mg four times daily. Amoxicillin in its formulation with clavulanic acid, Augmentin 500/125, orally four times daily, broadens ampicillin's spectrum to give activity against β-lactamase–producing staphylococci.

The aforementioned antimicrobials should be used in combination with hot packs at least 3 to 4 times daily. Topical antibiotics may be advisable in the case of a diseased cornea or if mucus discharge and ocular irritation exists. It is usually not possible to regurgitate pus through the canaliculi in acute dacryocystitis because of the edema of the tissues at the opening of the common canaliculus into the lacrimal sac. Attempts to probe or irrigate in the presence of acute dacryocystitis are hazardous. Special considerations that should prompt one to culture and Gram stain prior to initiating therapy include the ready availability of pus by gentle pressure over the sac, and the presence of a draining fistula or a virulent-appearing infection in an immunocompromised patient.

An infection that fails to respond, progressively worsens despite therapy, or appears to be pointing and ready to spontaneously drain should prompt one to perform either a needle aspiration of the sac or a stab incision followed by hot packs for 2 to 4 days. This allows another opportunity for microbiological studies to ensure that appropriate antibiotic therapy is being administered and will promote resolution of the acute infection in the majority of progressive cases. Routine incision and drainage is contraindicated because it may result in fistula formation. It is better, however, than spontaneous drainage and will help prevent progression to orbital cellulitis, orbital abscess, or even a septic cavernous sinus thrombosis, all of which carry a high morbidity.

The proper management of an acute dacryocystitis should include performing a DCR once inflammation has subsided. The technique for DCR is outlined in a recent review.[3] This can be performed as early as 10 to 14 days after the initiation of therapy. In cases of acute dacryocystitis that do not resolve on 7 to 14 days of antibiotic therapy, DCR may be necessary while inflammation is still present; however, it is technically much easier and safer to perform a DCR once inflammation has resolved. Some patients will have minimal epiphora between bouts of dacryocystitis, which makes it appear that a DCR is not necessary. However, one attack of dacryocystitis predisposes to future attacks that become more difficult to manage, and a DCR should be encouraged.

It must be remarked that in the case history given the management of this patient's tearing by intermittent office irrigation is inappropriate and ineffective except in the rare case of a partially obstructive dacryolith that may be irrigated through the nasolacrimal duct. Repeated office irrigation and especially nasolacrimal probing rarely result in any long-term benefit and may lead to permanent canalicular scarring.

In summary, this patient's management includes hot packs and the use of a systemic semisynthetic penicillin or cephalosporin for 10 to 14 days followed by a DCR. Aspiration or incision and drainage should be reserved for cases that worsen despite appropriate therapy or if spontaneous drainage appears imminent at the time of presentation.

References

1. McCord CD: The lacrimal drainage system, in Duane TD (ed): *Clinical Ophthalmology*, vol 4, Philadelphia, Harper & Row, Publishers, Inc, 1984, pp 1–25.
2. Doxanas MT, Anderson RL: *Clincial Orbital Anatomy*. Baltimore, Williams & Wilkins, 1984, pp 102–106.
3. Patrinely JR, Anderson RL: A review of lacrimal drainage surgery. *Ophthalmic Plastic Reconstruct Surg* 1986; 2:97–102.
4. Veirs ER: *Lacrimal Disorders, Diagnosis and Treatment*. St Louis, CV Mosby Co, 1976.
5. Seal DV, Barrett SP, McGill JI: Aetiology and treatment of acute bacterial infections of the external eye. *Br J Ophthalmol* 1982; 66:357–360.

Index